Arise Forth from the Couch...

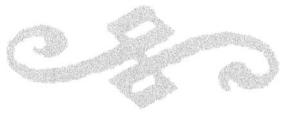

A Shakespearean Guide to Physical Fitness

Arise Forth from the Couch...[1]

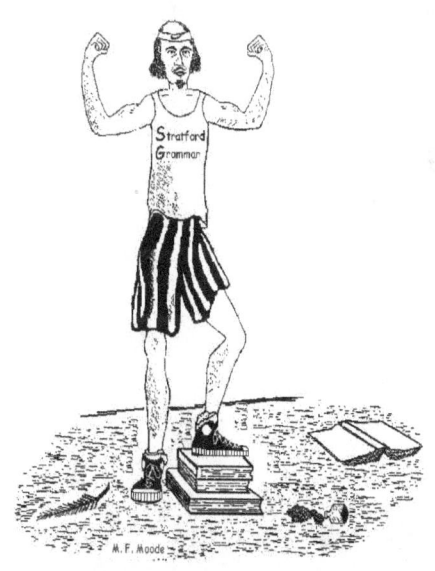

A Shakespearean Guide to Physical Fitness

Michael F. Moode

STEPHEN F. AUSTIN STATE UNIVERSITY PRESS
NACOGDOCHES ★ TEXAS

---

[1] King John Act III, Sc. IV

Copyright © 2012 by Stephen F. Austin State University
All rights reserved.
Printed in the United States of America.

No part of this book may be used or reproduced in any manner whatsoever without written permission except in the case of brief quotations embodied in critical articles or reviews.
PERMISSIONS:
Stephen F. Austin State University Press,
1936 North Street, LAN 203,
Nacogdoches, Texas, 75962.
sfapress@sfasu.edu

Book design: Brittany O'Sullivan
Editor: Laura Davis

LIBRARY OF CONGRESS CATALOGING-IN-PUBLICATION DATA

Moode, Michael F.
Arise Forth from the Couch
1st ed.
p. cm.
ISBN-13: 978-1-936205-60-8

First Edition: April 2012

To
Frank Andrews Moode

"He was a man, take him for all in all,
I shall not look upon his like again."

Hamlet: Act I, Sc. ii

For Mary and Marsha a special acknowledgment for their support, encouragement, assistance and inspiration.

"Beggar that I am, I am even poor in thanks..."

Hamlet: Act II, Sc. ii

Contents

Preface ❧ 9

I   Sweet Love! Sweet Lines! Sweet Life! ❧ 13

Why Physical Fitness? ❧ 13
- Elizabethan Toil and Modern Convenience ❧ 17
- Modern Lifestyle Dilemma ❧ 18
- Consequences of Inactive Lifestyles ❧ 19

II   More Things In Heaven And Earth ❧ 23

What Is Physical Fitness? ❧ 25
- Vigor, Alertness, and Energy ❧ 26
- Activity for Positive Physical Adaptations ❧ 27
- The Components of Physical Fitness ❧ 29
  - *Cardiorespiratory Endurance* ❧ 30
  - *Flexibility* ❧ 32
  - *Muscle Strength, Endurance, and Power* ❧ 33
  - *Body Composition* ❧ 34
- How Physical Fitness Training Works ❧ 38
  - *Overload* ❧ 38
  - *Progression* ❧ 39
  - *Specificity* ❧ 39

III   Dreams Are Indeed Ambition ❧ 41

Getting Fit ❧ 43
- Physical Activity and Exercise Approaches ❧ 43
- Purposeful Physically Active Lifestyles ❧ 44
- Sports and Games ❧ 45
- Exercise, Calisthenics, and Work-out Activities ❧ 47
- The Value of a Physically Active Lifestyle ❧ 48
- Elizabethan Activity and Lifestyles ❧ 49
- Activity Precautions and Preparation ❧ 50
  - *Duration* ❧ 52
  - *Frequency* ❧ 53
  - *Intensity* ❧ 54

IV To This Good Purpose 57
Exercise Activities 59
- Flexibility Exercises 60
- Muscle Properties 64
  - *Muscle Exercise and Contractions* 66
    - **Isometric Exercise** 66
    - **Isotonic Exercise** 66
    - **Isokinetic Exercise** 67
  - *Exercising for Muscular Strength* 68
  - *Exercising for Muscular Endurance* 69
- Walking 70
- Jogging 72
- Running 73
- Swimming 75
- Aquatic Exercises 77
- Cycling 79
- Stationary Exercise Bicycles 81
- Needful Counsel to Our Business 82
  - *Exercise Shoes and Fit Feet* 82
  - *Exercise Clothing* 84
- Final Thoughts 87

V My Life, My Joy, My Food 89
Nutrition, Diet, and Physical Fitness 91
- Digestion 95
- Knowledgeable Nutrition Choices 96
  - *Water* 98
  - *Fiber* 99
  - *Vitamins and Minerals* 100
- Energy Nutrients 102
  - *Carbohydrates* 102
  - *Protein* 103
  - *Fats* 104
- Eating Well—Nutritional Counsel 106
- Dieting, Physical Activity, and Weight Reduction 112

VI The Effect of This Good Lesson 117
Shakespearean Fitness Advice 119
- General Fitness Precepts 119
- Physical Activity Admonitions 122
- Nutrition, Diet and Body Composition 131

EPILOGUE 137
SELECTED BIBLIOGRAPHY 139

Preface

Shakespeare was, as Ben Jonson once commented, " **... not of an age, but for all time.**" His works present a universality of wisdom that is undeniable. His plays, poems, and sonnets are full of colorful, powerful language and essential insights on the human condition, including life, fitness, and health. By contrast, we who " **... live within this world ...** " [1] with our declining fitness and fading health may not even be for our *own time, let alone all time!* We are constantly reminded and cautioned by various medical authorities, government agencies, and our occasional inability to accomplish a simple physical task that "**. . . our little life [may soon] be rounded with a sleep.**" [2] This is directly attributable to our declining physical fitness and vigor.

In *Arise Forth from the Couch: A Shakespearean Guide to Physical Fitness,* the fundamental ideas, common truths as well as many of the misconceptions which underlie physical fitness are explained. To the general reader, the fitness professional, or anyone seeking a fundamental, entertaining, and novel presentation of physical fitness, this book is the perfect choice. Besides the lively, sometimes beautiful and often compelling prose which is used to accentuate various fitness concepts, the book acquaints the reader with essential views on the evolving characteristics, understanding, and appreciation for the concept of physical fitness in modern society as compared to Shakespeare's world.

Arise Forth from the Couch: A Shakespearean Guide to Physical Fitness begins by examining the nature and importance of physical fitness and reviews various activities commonly used today in order to achieve fitness goals. An underlying theme with regard to these basic concepts is the recognition that today we are aware of the need, benefit, and value of physical fitness, physical activity and a fitness lifestyle. However, in these " **... fair prosperous days ...** " [3] the attributes and knowledge are, as Hamlet might have described them, **"more honour'd in the breach than the observance."**[4] Subsequently, nutrition, diet, and weight management, are presented in a clear, non-academic, understandable manner. Finally, a variety of fitness truths, practices and mistaken beliefs are examined and explained.

1 King Richard II, Act V, Sc. III
2 The Tempest Act IV, Sc. I
3 King Richard III Act V, Sc. V
4 Hamlet Act I, Sc. IV

ARISE FORTH FROM THE COUCH: A SHAKESPEAREAN GUIDE TO PHYSICAL FITNESS

More than just a physical fitness how-to book, *Arise Forth from the Couch: A Shakespearean Guide to Physical Fitness* is brimming with basic explanations and solid advice to encourage exercise, training, and purposeful physically-active lifestyles. It is a book that the reader will enjoy rereading for motivation. Shakespeare's delightful, timeless, and robust language will hopefully inspire the reader to **"arise forth from the couch of lasting night"** [5] and pursue a physically fit and active lifestyle.

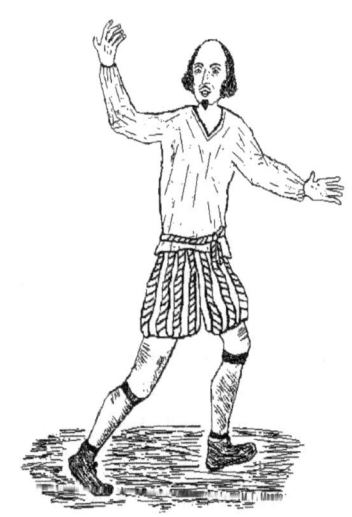

---

5   King John Act III, Sc. IV

Sweet Love! Sweet Lines! Sweet Life!

Chapter 1
Why Physical Fitness?
"Sweet love! sweet lines! sweet life!" [1]

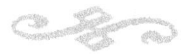

During the reign of England's Queen Elizabeth I (1558-1603) Shakespeare created some of the greatest thoughts and most incredible language that has ever been written. **"Words of so sweet breath composed."** [2] It was however, an era when life was demanding and physically difficult. Sickness and death were common features of everyday existence. Life expectancy was about forty years. Diseases were believed to be the result of an imbalance of the four humours. It was believed that these humours, black bile, blood, choler, and phlegm would, when in balance, lead to good health. When these humours were disproportionate or deficient, diseases such as **token'd pestilence**,[3] **quotidian**,[4] **ague**,[5] **dew-lapp'd throat**,[6] **serpigo**,[7] smallpox, tuberculosis, dysentery, or leprosy were the result. Additionally, health problems commonly associated with poor sanitation and food preparation, **devouring pestilence**,[8] and physically exhausting lifestyles were everyday realities.

> **"There's hell, there's darkness, there's the sulphurous pit,
> Burning, scalding, stench, consumption..."** [9]

London, the foremost city of Elizabethan England, was a disease and sanitation nightmare with raw sewage everywhere. Butchers regularly disposed of putrid and rotting carcasses in the streets, and all manner of debris and filth were commonplace. The smells, the sights, the squalor were all unbelievable in comparison to modern standards. In this environment, Shakespeare's Thane of Ross, a Scottish nobleman laments the situation in England:

---

1. The Two Gentlemen of Verona, Act I, Sc. III
2. Hamlet, Act III, Sc. I
3. plague - Antony and Cleopatra, Act III, Sc. X
4. malaria - King Henry V, Act IV, Sc. I
5. sweating sickness - King John Act V, Sc. III
6. goiter - The Tempest, Act III, Sc. III
7. skin eruptions - Measure For Measure, Act III, Sc. I
8. air pollution - King Richard II, Act I, Sc. III
9. King Lear, Act IV, Sc. VI

> "Alas poor country!
> Almost afraid to know itself. It cannot
> Be call'd our mother, but our grave; where nothing,
> But who knows nothing, is once seen to smile;
> Where sighs and groans and shrieks that rend the air
> Are made, not mark'd; where violent sorrow seems
> A modern ecstasy; the dead man's knell
> Is there scarce ask'd for who; and good men's lives
> Expire before the flowers in their caps,
> Dying or ere they sicken." [10]

In this life and health environment, another of Shakespeare's characters, Jaques, describes the sequences of Elizabethan life as a series of events or stages when he tells Rosalind's father, The Duke Senior, that:

> All the world's a stage,
> And all the men and women merely players:
> They have their exits and their entrances;
> And one man in his time plays many parts,
> His acts being seven ages. At first the infant,
> Mewling and puking in the nurse's arms.
> And then the whining school-boy, with his satchel
> And shining morning face, creeping like snail
> Unwillingly to school. And then the lover,
> Sighing like furnace, with a woeful ballad
> Made to his mistress' eyebrow. Then a soldier,
> Full of strange oaths and bearded like the pard,
> Jealous in honour, sudden and quick in quarrel,
> Seeking the bubble reputation
> Even in the cannon's mouth. And then the justice,
> In fair round belly with good capon lined,
> With eyes severe and beard of formal cut,
> Full of wise saws and modern instances;
> And so he plays his part. The sixth age shifts
> Into the lean and slipper'd pantaloon,
> With spectacles on nose and pouch on side,
> His youthful hose, well saved, a world too wide
> For his shrunk shank; and his big manly voice,
> Turning again toward childish treble, pipes
> And whistles in his sound. Last scene of all,
> That ends this strange eventful history,
> Is second childishness and mere oblivion,
> Sans teeth, sans eyes, sans taste, sans everything." [11]

---

10   MacBeth, Act IV, Sc. III
11   As You Like It, Act II, Sc. VII

This description, though 400 years old, portrays a view of life which includes distinct stages that in many respects are very much like the stages of life today. There is, however, an aspect of Shakespeare's description of life and life's sequences that was not even considered and utterly overlooked in Elizabethan times and virtually unrecognized and poorly understood until the twentieth century.

> **"There is a tide in the affairs of men,**
> **Which, taken at the flood, leads on to fortune;**
> **Omitted, all the voyage of their life**
> **Is bound in shallows and in miseries."** [12]

It is what today we might refer to as the quality of life or as Shakespeare might have described it **"life, with grace, health, beauty, honour."** [13] Superior "quality of life" is what everyone consciously or unconsciously desires. Good health, financial security, personal safety, and general feelings of well being all contribute to good living and a **"sweet life."**[14]

There was an underlying human attribute that was present, but not even acknowledged in Shakespeare's time and is even today often overlooked and neglected. This attribute involves the physiological functions and abilities which today we recognize and refer to as *physical fitness*. For virtually all of human history, humanity has survived and succeeded because we used the physical abilities with which we were born. Mankind gathered, hunted, farmed, grappled with nature, and physically worked at surviving. We did all of this instinctively with a fortunate evolutionary combination of brain, muscle, bone, and cardiovascular abilities in what Shakespeare might have referred to as the **"dignity of the whole body."** [15] The physical endeavors that humanity performed to survive were not always pleasant or easy but they were necessary and they were accomplished by humans who possessed and maintained their innate human physical abilities. Today we seem to have

> **". . forgone all custom of exercises."** [16]
> **"And by my body's action teach my mind. . ."** [17]

Of the body's muscles, bones, cardiovascular system, nervous tissues and brain we tend, **" ... for necessity of present life ... "** [18] to neglect and ignore all of these physiologic systems except perhaps for the brain. However, even the brain, **"neither savouring of**

12	Julius Caesar, Act IV, Sc. III
13	King Lear, Act I, Sc. I
14	King John, Act IV, Sc. III
15	Macbeth, Act V, Sc. I
16	Hamlet, Act II, Sc. II
17	Coriolanus, Act III, Sc. II
18	Othello, Act I, Sc. I

poetry, wit, nor invention" [19] "**. . . in the idle pleasures of these** [current] **day**[s]" [20] tends to deteriorate because of disregard and neglect.

> "**. . . we are not ourselves**
> **When nature, being oppress'd, commands the mind**
> **To suffer with the body.**" [21]

We do as little physical and mental work as we can, whenever we can! We are today well "**. . . conversant with ease and idleness.**" [22] It is not at all unusual for us to drive ourselves to a gym in order to work-out using various exercise machines that will help us exercise! Even in our present "**. . . fair prosperous days,**" [23] the ability to accomplish all matter of physical work remains an important aspect of mankind. This, even though we frequently seek, consciously or unconsciously, to avoid physical effort and activity and our "**. . . spirits are so married in conjunction with the participation of society that** [we] **... flock together in consent, like so many wild-geese.**" [24]

> "**Why, universal plodding poisons up**
> **The nimble spirits in the arteries . . .**" [25]

With regard to the **"sweet life"** it should be understood that physical fitness underlies all human functions. "**No less than life, with grace, health, beauty, honour**" [26] is improved by physically active lifestyles. Fitness is one of the best investments we can make toward the quality of our lives. Possessing health, vigor, looking toned, feeling well, and being in shape are rewards in and of themselves. There are more reasons to get and stay fit than there are fast food restaurants, miracle weight-loss formulas, and exotic new exercise programs. Recent studies have concluded that physical fitness may be more important in predicting life expectancy than any other single factor and may be the most effective anti-aging remedy that exists. Further, purposeful physical exercise that improves our physical fitness makes us feel and look better and can generally brighten our outlook on life. A physically active lifestyle can minimize the health problems associated with smoking, high blood pressure, high blood sugar and excess body fat. Thus, it becomes obvious that for individuals who are physically fit, good health, feelings of well being and the person's potential "**... for quiet days, fair issue and long life...** " [27] are enhanced.

19	Love's Labour's Lost, Act IV, Sc. II
20	King Richard III, Act I, Sc. I
21	King Lear, Act II, Sc. IV
22	King John, Act IV, Sc. III
23	King Richard III, Act V, Sc. V
24	King Henry IV, part II, Act V, Sc. I
25	Love's Labour's Lost, Act IV, Sc. III
26	King Lear, Act I, Sc. I
27	The Tempest, Act IV, Sc. I

Elizabethan Toil and Modern Convenience

**"Forspent with toil, as runners with a race,
I lay me down a little while to breathe;
For strokes received, and many blows repaid,
Have robb'd my strong-knit sinews of their strength,
And spite of spite needs must I rest awhile."** [28]

In Elizabethan England, in order to survive it was necessary to physically toil, **"... to grunt and sweat under a weary life..."** [29] Elizabethans desired moments and circumstances when they could take and enjoy **"... sweet repose and rest ..."** [30] In our trash-compacting, push-button, remote-controlled, elevator-riding, automatic-garage-door-opening, electric-pencil-sharpening, microwaveable lives we seek, pursue, and sometimes even pay good money to engage in *contrived* physical activity. We join health clubs and go to gymnasiums in order to improve, achieve, or maintain those physical attributes that our ancestors possessed naturally just to survive. Today we know that there are emotional, intellectual, and even vocational benefits to being fit and healthy and **". . . health shall live free and sickness freely die."** [31] Additionally, some people even acknowledge the physical aspect of their humanity and instead of engaging in daily regular purposeful activity **"... more honour'd in the breach than the observance"** [32] they seek fitness in health clubs, exercise spas and with exercise devices and gimmicks.

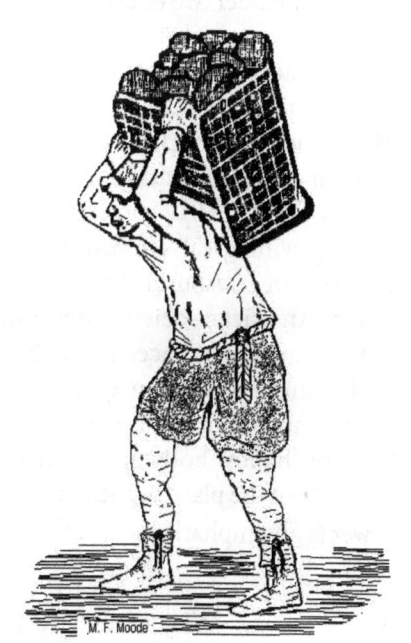

---

28 King Henry VI, part III, Act II, Sc. III
29 Hamlet, Act III Sc. I
30 Romeo and Juliet, Act II, Sc. I
31 All's Well That Ends Well, Act II, Sc. I
32 Hamlet, Act I, Sc. IV

Modern Lifestyle Dilemma

"O brave new world, That has such people in't." [33]

"... **Tis current in our land...**" [34] that people pursue their physical fitness and exercise with dogged determination. At least in their own minds! Physical activity and effort is pursued on a regular basis, every day, every other day, and perhaps for as much as an hour or two! "... **So much is the wonder in extremes.**" [35] Consider two, three, or four days of physical activity per week or even daily physical activity. Consider two or even three hours per activity session. Can these brief bouts of regular, measured activity really compensate for what our ancestors did everyday, all day, all the time? In today's "... **most brisk and giddy-paced times,**" [36] there are common and widespread misconceptions regarding physical fitness. It is not unusual to find people pursuing with great enthusiasm and commitment improper or unsound fitness goals. Women in modern American society often concentrate on their body's lean appearance. Men, by contrast, being equally misguided, concentrate on their muscle strength and their powerful appearing physiques.

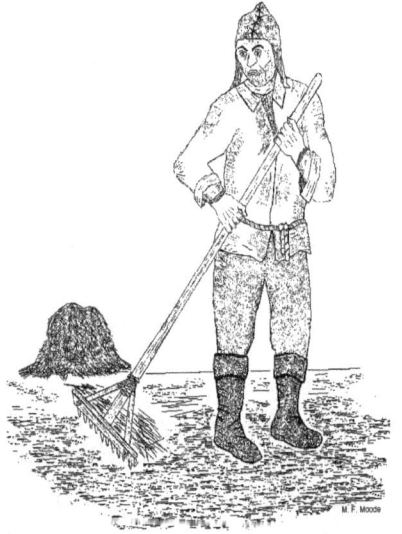

Do these shallow body appearance goals, and rationed or measured periods of physical activity, take the place of the constant physical effort and daily work of our ancestors? The answer is an emphatic no!

> "O heavens!
> Why does my blood thus muster to my heart,
> Making both it unable for itself,
> And dispossessing all my other parts
> Of necessary fitness?" [37]

The first and most obvious solution to modern fitness problems is the *regular* use of the body in physical activity. Walk, lift, carry, and work the body in the ways in which it was

---

33   The Tempest, Act V, Sc. I
34   King Richard Act II, Sc. III
35   King Henry VI, part III, Act III, Sc. II
36   Twelfth Night, Act II, Sc. IV
37   Measure for Measure, Act II, Sc. IV

meant to be used. We must understand that athletic performance and sports competition are recent phenomena in terms of human activities. Further, modern exercise programs, occasional or recreational sports participation, and the latest exercise devices do not necessarily qualify as meaningful physical activities. In fact, sports participation and competition can cause injury. This certainly is the case when it is performed irregularly and to the limit of a person's physical ability. Pushing the body too hard or too fast may result in harm, rather than contributing to fitness. Physical activity on a regular basis, wherever and whenever possible is a more desirable approach. It can and will contribute to the **"sweet life."**

> "And happily may your sweet self put on
> The lineal state and glory of the land!" [38]

Today we have more than doubled the Elizabethan life expectancy. These gains have resulted from better understanding of the causes and nature of diseases as well as superior medicines and improved personal and public health. Most of the acute infectious diseases that decimated humanity in Shakespeare's time are now well understood and can be cured or controlled. Unfortunately, the biggest health problems today are, in effect, self inflicted and caused by neglect and disregard of our bodies. Most of our lives are spent **"... living dully sluggardized at home,** [where we] **wear out** [our] **youth** [our health, our fitness, and our lives] **with shapeless idleness."** [39]

Consequences of Inactive Lifestyles

> "The fault, dear Brutus, is not in our stars, But in ourselves." [40]

𝔄 major contributor to this neglect certainly is the limited time we devote to physical activity and fitness.

> "Where wasteful time debateth with decay,
> To change your day of youth to sullied night ..." [41]

Sedentary lifestyles, automation, high-fat diets, and an abundance of leisure contribute to diminishing health and facilitate the sometimes spectacular decline of we modern **"... warriors for the working-day."** [42] **"... To the death, we will not move a foot ..."** [43] This physical deterioration has led today's clothing designers to produce all manner

38	King John, Act V, Sc. VII
39	The Two Gentlemen of Verona, Act I, Sc. I
40	Julius Caesar, Act I, Sc. II
41	Sonnet XV
42	King Henry V, Act IV, Sc. III
43	Love's Labour's Lost, Act V, Sc. II

of loose fitting styles, extremely stretchy fabrics and such remarkable clothing advances as hidden padded waist bands capable of incredible expansion! Similarly, furniture manufacturers have had to redesign their products to hold our larger body dimensions. **"No longer** [just] **from head to foot ... [**but also**] from hip to hip..."** [44] chairs, beds and other common items of furniture are routinely being redesigned, strengthened and reinforced to accommodate **"the thick rotundity o' ..."** [45] our bodies which have made us **"... spherical like ... globe**[s]**."** [46]

"Nothing but sit and sit, and eat and eat!" [47]

Additionally, these factors contribute to the prevalence of chronic illnesses that are so common today and were virtually unknown in Shakespeare's time. Health problems like cardiovascular disease, hypertension, and diabetes were nonexistent 400 years ago. Cardiovascular disease and cancer have replaced tuberculosis and pneumonia as the two leading causes of death. Perhaps as much as a third of the modern American population will develop cancer while another third will suffer cardiovascular diseases. While these diseases primarily affect adults, they are often the end result of behaviors begun in childhood. For example, it has been documented that abnormally high levels of cholesterol are already present in children under the age of ten.

"They are now starved for want of exercise. . ." [48]

Due to technology and our many modern labor saving devices, physical activity is no longer a normal part of our daily lives. **"He stirreth not, he moveth not ..."** [49] We may find ourselves like Barnardine, in *Measure Fore Measure*, who, being imprisoned, is described by the Provost as unconcerned by death having lived and neglected his life in a manner which was . . .

"... careless, reckless, and fearless of what's past, present, or to come; insensible of mortality, and desperately mortal." [50]

This description of Barnardine might well be applied to many of us today. In modern society we know much more about disease, healthy living, exercise, and physical fitness, however we continue to live increasingly sedentary if not stationary lives.

44	The Comedy of Errors, Act III, Sc. II
45	King Lear, Act III, Sc. II
46	King Lear, Act III, Sc.II
47	The Taming of the Shrew Act V, Sc. II
48	Pericles, Prince of Tyre, Act I, Sc. IV
49	Romeo and Juliet, Act II, Sc. I
50	Measure For Measure, Act IV, Sc. II

"Alas, our frailty is the cause, not we!" [51]

The human body has always been capable of adapting to practically any level of physical activity and exertion. In our present **"... doleful days,"** [52] the level of activity to which our bodies adapt to is minimally low, of short duration, and usually not very intense. Stated another way—we are not demanding much from our bodies and certainly not getting much back!

"... the more it is wasted the sooner it wears." [53]

Our Elizabethan ancestors, because of the physical demands of life and necessity of regular manual labor, probably were more physically fit than we are today. **"There is no virtue like necessity."** [54] The value of physical fitness is both physical and mental, immediate and long term. Physical fitness can be like **"... a medicine that's able to breathe life into a stone, quicken a rock, and make you dance canary** [55] **with spritely fire and motion..."** [56]

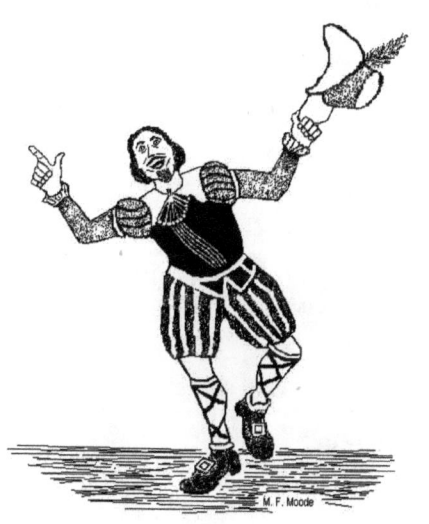

Finally, being physically fit makes it easier to accomplish our **"... barren tasks, too hard to keep."** [57] It facilitates the presence of reserve energy for emergencies, and it helps us look and feel better. Fitness enhances the body's resistance to chronic diseases and helps us protect ourselves more effectively against acute diseases. Fit people can and do maintain their physical and mental well-being throughout their lives. They are healthy, happier, live longer, and enjoy their lives more than their non-fit friends. **"It is silliness to live when to live is torment ..."** [58]

"Heaven, from thy endless goodness, send prosperous life, long, and ever happy ..." [59]

51	Twelfth Night Act II, Sc. II
52	King Henry IV, part II, Act II, Sc. IV
53	King Henry IV, part I, Act II, Sc. IV
54	King Richard II, Act I, Sc. III
55	A lively old French dance
56	All's Well That Ends Well, Act II, Sc. I
57	Love's Labour's Lost, Act I, Sc. I
58	Othello, Act I, Sc. III
59	King Henry VIII, Act V, Sc. V

More Things in Heaven and Earth

Chapter II
WHAT IS PHYSICAL FITNESS?

"There are more things in heaven and earth, Horatio, Than are dreamt of in your philosophy." [1]

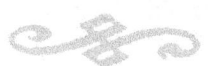

The exact nature of physical fitness is widely misunderstood. In modern society, as previously stated, women often associate physical fitness with weight loss and an attractive slim shape. Men commonly focus on muscular development and an athletic physique.

"beautified with goodly shape." [2]

Others believe that physical fitness is the ability to engage in and perform in an athletic or sports environment—

"Some say thy grace is youth and gentle sport" [3]

And still others view fitness as feelings of vigor or freedom from disease—

"lusty, young, and cheerly drawing breath." [4]

There is an element of accuracy in each of these views but taken individually, they miss the true nature and importance of physical fitness.

---

1   Hamlet, Act I, Sc. V
2   The Two Gentlemen of Verona, Act IV, Sc. I
3   Sonnet XCVI
4   King Richard, Act I, Sc. III

Arise Forth from the Couch: A Shakespearean Guide to Physical Fitness

Vigor, Alertness, and Energy

"The rich advantage of good exercise" [5]

When considering fitness, some might include such attributes as emotional well being, intellectual aptitude, spiritual awareness, social abilities, as well as the above-mentioned physical qualities. These, however, fall appropriately in the area of wellness and are far beyond the fundamental concept of physical fitness.

"Each hath his place and function" [6]

Physical fitness is measured by the functional performances of the cardiorespiratory system, muscle strength, muscle endurance, joint flexibility and body composition. **"Here lies thy heart, thy sinews, and thy bone."** [7] Additionally, physical performance stress tests evaluate the body's ability to respond and adapt to moderately intense levels of physical effort. If we are able to respond favorably to a stress test, then we would be considered to be physically fit. To most of us, physical fitness is regarded as the ability to comfortably get through **"the incessant care and labour"** [8] of our daily lives. This being accomplished, we should feel well enough and have enough energy to deal with unexpected physical demands, should they arise. Additionally, at the end of the day the physically fit individual should feel well enough, vigorous enough, and possess sufficient energy to enjoy recreational activities of a physical nature, such as golf, a walk, or a swim.

"you are now well enough: how came you thus recovered?" [9]

Stated another way, a person is physically fit when he or she can meet both the ordinary as well as the unexpected demands of daily life efficiently and effectively while still possessing sufficient vigor at the end of the working day for *recreational* physical activities. In a practical sense, not only are most of us incapable of meeting physical demands of life but in modern society these demands are relatively low. **"And every day that comes comes to decay"** [10]

---

5   King John, Act IV, Sc. II
6   King Henry, VI, part I, Act I, Sc. I
7   Troilus and Cressida, Act V, Sc. VIII
8   King Henry IV, part II, Act IV, Sc. IV
9   Othello, Act II, Sc. III
10   Cymbeline Act I, Sc. V

Activity for Positive Physical Adaptations

"Our bodies are our gardens, to the which our wills are gardeners" [11]

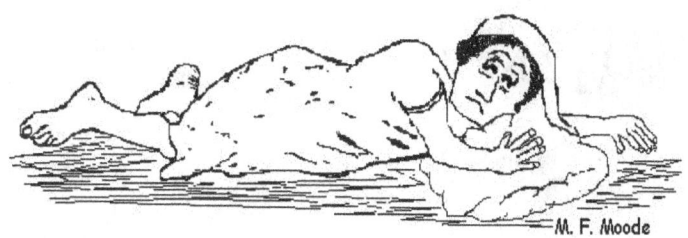

Consider **"how weary, stale, flat and unprofitable,"** [12] daily jobs, businesses, and labors are in terms of physical exertion. Most people's "work" today usually involves papers that need to be shuffled, items that need to be sold or purchased, meetings that need to be attended, desk work routines that need to be accomplished, phones, FAXs, e-mails and sitting in front of computers. In the most vigorous modern occupations, an engine or mechanical appliance must be supervised and operated and then, following work and a suitable amount of television viewing we, "**... with a body fill'd and vacant mind ...**"[13] "**... weary with toil ... haste**" [14] to bed.

If we accept the preceding stereotypical description of modern life and any of the preceding definitions of fitness, in essence everyone could be classified as being physically fit. The office worker, salesperson, teacher, merchant, truck driver almost everybody gets through their daily responsibilities and yet remains capable of running up a flight of stairs when late for an appointment, a class, or a meeting. **"Thou know'st thy country's strength and weakness."** [15] Additionally, that same person may engage in physical recreational activities if not daily at least on weekends, engaging in a round of golf, a little tennis, a bit of touch football, a game of softball for fun, recreation, or exercise. **"He is given to sports, to wildness and much company."** [16]

11	Othello, Act I, Sc. III
12	Hamlet, Act I, Sc. II
13	King Henry V, Act IV, Sc. I
14	Sonnett XXVII.
15	Coriolanus, Act IV, Sc. V
16	Julius Caesar, Act II, Sc. I

These modern lifestyle activities are not as intense or regular as the physical activity of Elizabethans. **"The incessant care and labour"** [17] of life was considerably more physical and vigorous. The hunter, farmer, and tradesman all plied their trades with little or no labor-saving or mechanical help. **"For hunting was his daily exercise."** [18] They lifted, carried, and moved from place to place by the power of their own human abilities. Therefore, the preceding definition is probably not sufficient when we consider modern lifestyles.

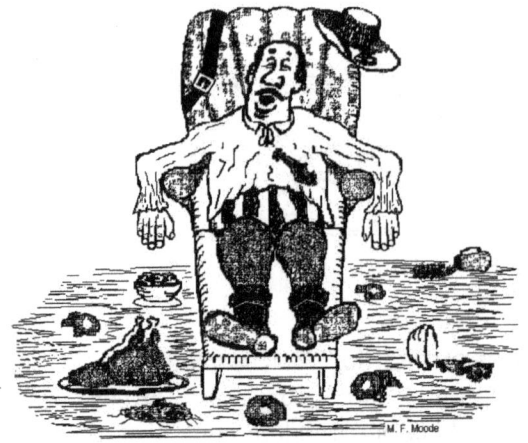

"Now is my day's work done; i'll take good breath" [19]

A more appropriate description of physical fitness has been verbalized by The American Medical Association. The AMA views physical fitness as the ability of the body to respond and adapt favorably to the demands and stresses of physical work, exertion, and activity.

"And we must take the current when it serves" [20]

The more often and vigorously that we challenge our muscles, bones, heart, lungs, blood, and the body in general, the more fit they will remain. However, the opposite is likewise true. The fewer physical demands we place on our bodies, the more likely **"those organs** [are to develop] **... deceptious function."** [21]

"See how the blood is settled in his face." [22]

When our bodies do not regularly engage in physical activity and few physical demands are placed on our physiological systems, they begin to deteriorate. The negative effects of physical inactivity on our bodies has long been recognized and understood.

**"What is a man,
If his chief good and market of his time
Be but to sleep and feed? "** [23]

17	King Henry IV, part II, Act IV, Sc. IV
18	King Henry VI, part III, Act IV, Sc. VI
19	Troilus and Cressida Act V, Sc. VIII
20	Julius Caesar, Act Iv, Sc. III
21	Troilus and Cressida, Act V, Sc. II
22	King Henry VI, part II, Act III, Sc. II
23	Hamlet, Act IV, Sc. IV

Neglect, **"with his stealing steps, hath clawed me in his clutch."** [24] Neglected bones lose their density, joints become stiff, muscles become weaker and smaller, energy levels diminish while body fat accumulates, the heart becomes weaker, blood vessels clogged, and circulatory system inefficient.

"He is deformed, crooked, old and sere[25]
Ill-faced, worse bodied, shapeless everywhere" [26]

To preserve or improve physical fitness, we must maintain reasonable levels of activity, work, movement, and motion throughout our entire lifetime.

"The want is but to put those powers in motion
That long to move." [27]

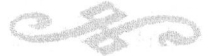

THE COMPONENTS OF PHYSICAL FITNESS

"Does not our life consist of the four elements?" [28]

The preceding views of physical fitness may be more easily understood and simplified by looking at the four different components, or attributes of the body that underlie and facilitate physical fitness. That is, physical fitness is most easily understood by examining its constituent parts. According to virtually all fitness experts, the components of physical fitness include: (1) cardiorespiratory endurance, (2) normal joint flexibility, (3) appropriate levels of muscular strength and endurance, and (4) a body composition that reflects a suitable and desirable ratio between lean-body mass to fat-body mass. Everyone should be concerned with the degree to which these individual components are present.

---

24   Hamlet, Act V, Sc. I
25   Dried up; withered
26   The Comedy of Errors Act IV, Sc. II
27   Cymbeline, Act IV, Sc. III
28   Twelfth Night, Act II, Sc. III

Cardiorespiratory Endurance

**"a good heart, ... , is the sun and the moon;
or, rather, the sun, and not the moon;
for it shines bright and never changes,
but keeps his course truly."** [29]

What causes weariness of arms, legs, spirit, and the body generally? Fatigue results from the body's inability to produce enough chemical energy for the muscles to continue their work.

**"universal plodding poisons up
The nimble spirits in the arteries,
As motion and long-during action tires
The sinewy vigour"** [30]

The chemical source of energy used by the muscles, as well as all other cells in the body, is called adenosinetriphoshpate (ATP). The body's ability to produce the greatest quantity of this energy-rich compound in the most efficient manner occurs when there is ample oxygen and sufficient nutrients present in the circulatory system.

"breath and blood" [31]

Cardiorespiratory endurance or aerobic fitness is the ability of the cardiovascular and respiratory systems to adapt to, as well as recover from life's stress and physical activity. It is considered the most important component of physical fitness. Cardiorespiratory endurance or aerobic fitness is present when **"our hearts are in the trim"** [32] we possess **"sensible and nimble lungs"** [33] and **"affections and warm youthful blood."** [34] That is, the ability of the body to take in, absorb, transport, and deliver oxygen as well as nutrients to working muscles for long periods of time. Additionally, the removal of carbon dioxide and other metabolic wastes during physical activity, as well as during recovery following physical activity, are essential aspects of cardiorespiratory endurance.

"More would I, but my lungs are wasted so" [35]

29	King Henry V, Act V, Sc. II
30	Love's Labour's Lost, Act IV, Sc. III
31	King Lear, Act II, Sc. IV
32	King Henry V, Act IV, Sc. III
33	The Tempest, Act II, Sc. I
34	Romeo and Juliet, Act II, Sc. V
35	King Henry IV, part II, Act IV, Sc. V

If we neglect our cardiovascular system it becomes inefficient and incapable of producing adequate amounts of the body's chemical energy, ATP. This ATP energy deficiency is usually caused because not enough **"healthsome air breathes in"** [36] and therefore **"through all thy veins shall run a cold and drowsy humour."** [37] When the cells' access to sufficient oxygen supplies is inadequate their ability to produce energy is impeded. Disuse, neglect, and decreased demands on these systems are commonly the cause of the decline of cells' ability to produce the body's chemical energy.

"till thou hast worn out thy pump" [38]

Cardiorespiratory or aerobic ability is, in its simplest sense, the mechanism by which the body produces chemical energy in the presence of adequate amounts of oxygen. Physical activity that lasts a long time and is moderately intense or vigorous will meet its energy needs through aerobic physiological processes. During these long duration, moderately intense physical activities the muscles demand and thereby force the body's various physiological systems to take-in, transport, and furnish oxygen and nutrients in order to support and continue the physical activity and muscle effort.

"a good heart's worth gold" [39]

Aerobic exercise works your heart improving its function and strength as well as your circulatory system facilitating **"this confine of blood and breath"** [40] improving their capacity and efficiency. It works the respiratory system contributing to its effectiveness as well as the body's other physiological systems.

"A light heart lives long." [41]

Basic activities like walking, carrying, and lifting are all highly aerobic and contribute to the maintenance of the cardiorespiratory system. Aerobic activities are usually natural, useful and involve the movements which most people have been performing throughout all human history just to survive. Physical activities like running, swimming, weight lifting, and cycling have become the activities that many people in modern society choose to engage in to compensate for their lack of the more natural forms of aerobic, cardiorespiratory activity. Generally, cardiorespiratory endurance or aerobic fitness is essential to high level fitness and wellness as well as a long and healthy life.

"Health and long life to you" [42]

36	Romeo and Juliet, Act IV, Sc. III
37	Romeo and Juliet, Act IV, Sc. I
38	Romeo and Juliet, Act II, Sc. IV
39	King Henry IV, part II, Act II, Sc. IV
40	King John, Act IV, Sc. II
41	Love's Labour's Lost, Act V, Sc. II
42	King Henry IV part II, Act V, Sc. III

Flexibility

> "wretch, whose fever-weaken'd joints
> Like strengthless hinges, buckle under life ... " [43]

Flexibility exercises are commonly associated with and seen in sport warm-ups, athletic performances and competitive activities. Flexibility is the ability of muscles, bones, and joints to move through the greatest possible range of motion. Flexibility is not a general trait but rather it is joint specific. Thus, a person may possess excellent range of motion in a joint on one side of the body and less of a range in the corresponding joint on the other side or in other joints.

> "If thou neglect'st or dost unwillingly
> What I command, I'll rack thee with old cramps,
> Fill all thy bones with aches, make thee roar
> That beasts shall tremble at thy din" [44]

Regular and useful physical activity contributes to bone integrity and joint flexibility. Conversely, our sedentary lifestyles, **"all men idle, all; And women too,"** [45] may lead to the loss of bone density and joint functions, thereby reducing flexibility. **"His weary joints would gladly rise, I know."** [46] The maintenance of flexibility or its improvement should not be the exclusive domain of athletics and sport activities. It should be a constant and regular part of our daily lives. Flexibility exercise and activities, performed regularly, would enhance and facilitate virtually all of our everyday tasks. Daily activities like getting dressed, rising from a chair, reaching up for an object on a shelf, or turning the head to look backward while driving are all easier to accomplish if we possess flexibility.

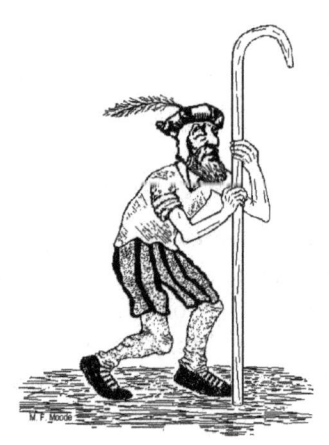

> **"Youth is nimble, age is lame"** [47]

43	King Henry IV, part II, Act I, Sc. I
44	The Tempest, Act I, Sc. II
45	The Tempest, Act II, Sc. I
46	King Richard II, Act V, Sc. III
47	Sonnet XII

As we age, diminishing flexibility, particularly of the back and hips may contribute to difficulty with everyday movements, lead to poor posture, back pain, and detract from people's ability to engage in useful physical activity.

"Thy bones are hollow; impiety has made a feast of thee" [48]

The range of motion of a joint is determined by a variety of factors. Perhaps the most obvious is the shape of the bones that form the joint. Excessive body fat which may be under the skin and around a joint or joints can hinder and limit a joint's range of motion. In a similar manner, though far less common especially with our modern lifestyles, large muscles and tight tendons may be factors that limit flexibility. In the final analysis, our sedentary lifestyles, joint neglect and disease are perhaps the most significant and immediate causes that **"shorten up their sinews"** [49] and result in reduced **"vigour of bone,"** [50] joint flexibility, and losses in range of motion.

"His weary joints would gladly rise . . . ." [51]

With appropriate flexibility training exercises, joint range of motion can be maintained or enhanced. This does not mean that flexibility will be improved at the same rate for everyone. Generally, the older you are, the longer it will take to regain or achieve flexibility.

"His legs are legs for necessity, not for flexure." [52]

Though flexibility can be improved relatively quickly in comparison to other fitness components it is best to approach enhanced flexibility systematically and patiently.

Muscle Strength, Endurance, and Power

" ... my want of strength, my sick heart shows, that I must yield my body to the earth ..." [53]

Muscular strength is the ability of muscles to produce force. Muscular endurance, a separate muscle property, is the ability of a muscle to sustain or repeat contractions over a period of time. With reasonable levels of muscular strength and endurance people today should be able to achieve efficient movement, maintain desirable postures, engage comfortably in purposeful physical activity and ultimately enjoy fitness, health and wellness. Power, is a third property of skeletal muscles and is closely associated with and

---

48	Measure For Measure, Act I, Sc. 2
49	The Tempest, Act IV, Sc. I
50	Troilus and Cressida, Act III, Sc. III
51	King Richard II, Act V, Sc. III
52	Troilus and Cressida, Act II, Sc. III
53	King Henry VI, Part III, Act V, Sc. II

dependent on strength. It is the ability of a muscle to produce force *quickly*. Power is a property of muscles that throughout most of human history was only incidentally and indirectly valued. In modern times, power has emerged as an essential part of competitive sport, games, and athletic events.

"He has his health and ampler strength indeed" [54]

When muscles of the body possess strength, they are capable of producing force. The more strength the more force. Force is created by converting chemical fuel, ATP, into mechanical energy which moves the bones. When muscles are capable of producing force a person is able to push, pull, lift, work, move, exercise or play. The term force, in the context of muscular exertion, is synonymous with strength. Muscle endurance is a separate and distinct property from strength. It is the ability of a muscle to repeat or sustain a muscle contraction. Endurance requires the same chemical energy, ATP, as strength. However, endurance requires continual efficient physiological performance, function and support from the body's circulatory, respiratory, and digestive systems, in order to continue and maintain the muscles' endurance capacity.

Muscular strength and endurance are essential for good posture, personal appearance, numerous life activities and physical fitness. The person with adequate levels of muscle strength and endurance should experience less fatigue.

Body Composition

"The outward composition of his body" [55]

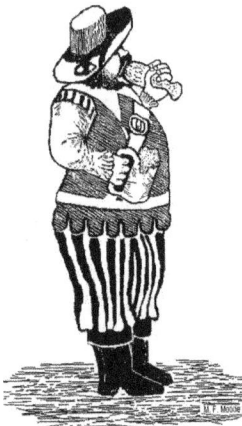

Body composition refers to the various physiological systems and the amount of tissue that constitutes the human body. From a fitness perspective and in its simplest sense, the human body is composed of muscles, bones, specialized tissues and organs, and fat. The non-fat components of the body are referred to as lean body tissue or lean body mass. That part of the body which is not classified as lean body mass is body fat.

"In thy fats our cares be drown'd" [56]

Body fat cells are normal, desirable, and are present in all humans at birth. These cells are wonderfully efficient energy storage

---

54   The Winter's Tale, Act IV, Sc. IV
55   King Henry VI, part I, Act II, Sc. III
56   Antony and Cleopatra, Act II, Sc. VII

warehouses that we, in modern society, begin filling with surplus and unused energy during childhood and continue filling them throughout our lives. Is it any wonder that over the years we **"grew by our feeding to so great a bulk."**[57] It is body fat cells that are overstuffed with surplus energy that we wear under our skin that is the greatest concern to our vigor, fitness, and function. When body fat cells are excessively filled they negatively affect circulation, respiration, feelings of vigor and wellness, and cause diminished health.

"He's fat, and scant of breath" [58]

Like flexibility, it is not the passage of time that necessarily makes a person **"a gross fat man."** [59] Rather, it is neglect and lifestyle eating habits. It is the way we live our lives!

"If the cook help to make the gluttony, you help to make the diseases." [60]

Relative to the fat under our skin, there is a common misconception that two types of depot body fat exist. These two types of fat are believed to be regular body fat and cellulite.

"dimples of his chin and cheek" [61]

Cellulite is assumed to be the "dimply," "lumpy," or "cottage cheese" textured type of fat that gives skin an unpleasant unattractive texture. In reality, however, this is just *body fat*. This being the case, all of those creams, massage therapy treatments, and special diet supplements that claim to eliminate cellulite are just scams. They are products and procedures that claim to eliminate a substance that does not exist. In fact, the fat under the skin is just like fat anywhere else in the body it has just "clumped" together and therefore gives skin an unnatural and unattractive appearance.

It is a widely held yet subtle belief that body fat, especially excessive fat, is ugly, abhorrent, and undesirable.

" ... to be fat be to be hated" [62]

Another aspect of body composition that most modern American women possess to varying degrees is a negative self image of themselves. They believe that they are too fat and would be much happier and more attractive if they were just thinner. In " ... **the thick rotundity o'** [today's] **world**" [63] there may be an element of truth in the belief that we are too fat, whether man or woman. However, among young girls this belief in and feeling of excessive body fat becomes more deeply held as these young girls grow into women whether they are fat or not.

---

57   King Henry IV, part I, Act V, Sc. I
58   Hamlet, Act V, Sc. II
59   King Henry IV, part I, Act II, Sc. IV
60   Henry IV, Part II, Act II, Sc. IV
61   The Winter's Tale, Act II, Sc. III
62   King Henry IV, part I, Act II, Sc. IV
63   King Lear, Act III, Sc. II

Additionally, there exists a vague notion that thinness is associated with beauty, success and self-control. Conversely, excess body fat or obesity is commonly associated with poor self control, ugliness and a lack of intelligence.

"beauty is bought by judgement of the eye." [64]

These same women, and society generally, are obsessed and preoccupied with fat—real or imagined and view themselves as " **... spread of late into goodly bulk."** [65]

The fat portion of the body should be viewed and evaluated in terms of its percentage of fat relative to the total weight of all other body components. Generally, it is recommended that men's bodies should possess approximately fifteen percent fat relative to total body weight. For women it is recommended that the percent body fat be approximately twenty percent of the total body weight. The higher percentage recommended for women is directly related to fertility and reproductive differences and is essential for good health. The problem today is that women have come to believe that with a skinnier, virtually fat free body their lives, romance, personal fulfillment, every aspect of existence will be improved and they will live merrily as **"lean, raw-boned rascals!"** [66]

"Lord, what fools these mortals be!" [67]

This view, that we will have better lives and be more attractive is so deeply imbedded in our collective subconscious that we frequently seek beauty and fulfillment through poor nutrition, unsound exercising, as well as drastically reduced and unhealthy eating.

"Forbear, and eat no more." [68]

To adjust and change body composition it is widely believed that the use of localized exercise, mechanical massage, or vibrating devices can diminish excessive fat. It is clear that these beliefs and practices are unsound and ineffective. If reduction of **"the spot of this enforced cause"** [69] were possible, people could simply do sit-ups to reduce fat on the abdomen, biceps curls to slim the arms, walk to diminish fat on the legs, and chew gum to reduce a chubby face. There is no evidence to support the idea that if you exercise a particular area of your body, you will reduce the excess fat in that region. Regular purposeful physical activity and reasonably vigorous and continuous exercises that involve large muscle groups, at a moderate intensity for long periods of time, do contribute to losses of fat. This fat reduction occurs in a general way throughout the whole body. Weight training exercises, along with aerobic activities benefit the cardiorespiratory system and provide the best means for diminishing fat. It is important to remember that physical activity and exercises intended to reduce body fat must be accompanied by reduced caloric intake.

64		Love's Labour's Lost, Act II, Sc. I
65		The Winter's Tale, Act II, Sc. I
66		King Henry VI, part I, Act I, Sc. II
67		A Midsummer Night's Dream, Act III, Sc. II
68		As You Like It, Act II, SC. VII
69		King John, Act V, Sc. II

It is virtually impossible to expend sufficient energy through exercise to compensate for excessive eating.

"'tis sweating labour" [70]

Another unsound and yet common behavior relative to body composition is the practice pursued by many of overheating the body in order to quickly lose excess weight by sweating it off. **"With such an agony, he sweat extremely."** [71] Exercising in hot, humid weather or exercising while wearing a rubber sweat suit or even more foolishly, *sitting* in saunas or steam baths are practices widely believed to quickly contribute to weight loss through profuse sweating.

"With that which melteth fools" [72]

These behaviors may reduce the reading on a scale but the reduction is sadly temporary. The weight that is lost through these practices has very little to do with body fat and is primarily the result of fluid loss. This fluid loss, if it takes place while exercising, can be life threatening. This, because a rubber sweat suit, excess clothing, or intense activity during hot humid weather will not allow the heat produced during exercise to dissipate from the body.

"Fie! this is hot weather, gentlemen" [73]

Sweating itself is not a hazard—it is a healthy and a normal means of maintaining optimal body temperature. The evaporation of sweat is the primary means by which the body eliminates heat.

"beads of sweat have stood upon thy brow" [74]

When you wear a rubber suit, the sweat does not evaporate. This causes body temperature to become higher than normal. This will cause an excessive loss of body fluids, reduced blood volume, minerals are flushed out through the skin, and the body temperature rises. Fluids and weight lost from this type of exercise will be replaced in a short period of time —certainly within hours as you eat and drink. The key point is that excessive sweating is unsound and unwise behavior for changing body composition. Water and sweat contain no calories, and unhealthy body composition will only be changed by reducing body fat and by enhancing lean body mass through a sound and safe exercise approach.

"they would melt me out of my fat" [75]

---

70 Antony and Cleopatra, Act I, Sc. III
71 King Henry, Act VIII, Sc. I
72 Julius Caesar, Act III, Sc. I
73 King Henry IV, part II, Act III, Sc. II
74 King Henry IV, part I, Act II, Sc. III
75 Merry Wives of Windsor, Act IV, Sc. V

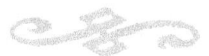

How Physical Fitness Training Works

"To give full growth to that which still doth grow" [76]

Physiologically, "training" is simple. Training is the means through which the body learns to *respond and adapt* to the physical demands. Whether through sports, exercise, a physically active lifestyle or a combination of all three, the body becomes more effective at adapting and becomes better able to cope with physical demands. The more physically active our lives are, the better and more likely positive physical abilities and adaptations will result. We should keep in mind, however, that not all physical demands and efforts are positive and desirable. Excessive, severe, or inappropriate physical demands may result in injury, pain, or impairment and hinder physical function and detract from fitness.

"The injuries that to myself I do" [77]

A physically active lifestyle is a good place to start a fitness program. Then, in order to achieve even higher levels of fitness, various exercises, activities and drills may be included. When planning and performing these supplemental physical activities, there are three extremely important principles to consider which are related to the physiological phenomena of training. **"These three lead on this preparation"** [78] they are the overload principle, progression, and specificity of training.

Overload

"he feels no pain, the one lacking the burden" [79]

In order to improve physical fitness, we need to work each of the fitness components slightly beyond their usual working limits. We must exceed our usual physiological barrier to achieve and set a new improved limit. Generally, it is recommended that we work at an intensity level that is sufficiently vigorous and lasts long enough to overload a component of fitness beyond its normal level. We must approach or exceed physiological fitness barriers and thereby bring about improved fitness. **"Exceed the common or be caught."**[80] Appropriately vigorous activity sessions every other day will make it more likely that physical fitness levels will improve. That is, you cannot hoard activity or exercise for use on weekends only or just once in a while. Regularity is essential.

---

76   Sonnet CXV
77   Sonnet LXXXVIII
78   Coriolanus, Act I, Sc. II
79   As you Like It, Act III, Sc. II
80   Coriolanus, Act IV, Sc. I

Progression

"A thousand hearts are great within my bosom: Advance our standards" [81]

To improve any of the components of physical fitness we must gradually make our physical activity more vigorous. We should begin with easy activity, **"wisely and slow; they stumble that run fast."** [82] Gradually increase intensity **"thereby to see the minutes how they run."** [83] Additionally, the frequency and duration of activity should progressively increase in order to enhance fitness levels.

"Give you advancement. Be it your charge ... " [84]

Some activities can be used to improve more than one of the fitness components. In addition to increasing cardiorespiratory endurance, jogging can improve muscular endurance in the legs, may be a positive factor on bones and joints, and diminish body fat. Swimming develops the arm, shoulder and chest muscles. If you select the proper activities, it is possible to fit parts of your muscular endurance work-out into your cardiorespiratory work-out and save time.

Specificity

"Be wisely definite" [85]

Specificity is the recognition that whatever physiological adaptations that take place as a result of training will be in direct and specific response to the demands that are experienced. Stated another way, physical activity only improves the fitness component that you work. **"In brief, sir, study what you most affect."** [86] Fitness training or physical training improvements of any kind are precise and definite. Training is NOT a general phenomenon. To improve a particular component you must work that component. Adaptations result directly from and in response to whatever activity is undertaken. Therefore, lift heavy weights with the arm muscles (the demand)—get *stronger* in the arm muscles that are worked (the adaptation).

"a good-limbed fellow; young, strong" [87]

---

81 King Richard III, Act V, Sc. III
82 Romeo and Juliet, Act II, Sc. III
83 King Henry VI, part III, Act II, Sc. V
84 King Henry IV, part II, Act V Sc. V
85 Cymbeline, Act I, Sc. VI
86 The Taming of the Shrew, Act I, Sc. I
87 King Henry IV, part II, Act III, Sc. II

Lift light weights with the arms (the demand)—develop *endurance* in the arm muscles that are worked.

" ... all your strict preciseness come to this" [88]

Strength is not endurance and endurance is not strength (specificity). Strength training results in specific strength changes. This very simple and narrow example should be understood by anyone who desires to improve or maintain physical fitness. The components that constitute physical fitness must be worked in specific ways so that the desired adaptations are achieved.

Finally, we must understand that no single physical activity, exercise, or sport is perfect for improving or maintaining physical fitness. We should engage in different types of physical activities as well as change the frequency, intensity, and duration of our usual activities. Living actively and participating in a variety of physical activities facilitates the acquisition of fitness. Additionally, varied activities help us avoid feelings of depression, training plateaus, and can minimize potential risks of overuse injury which might result if we engaged in only one type of exercise or activity.

---

88   King Henry VI, part I, Act V, Sc. IV

Dreams Are Indeed Ambition

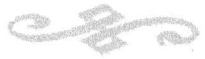

Chapter III
GETTING FIT
"dreams indeed are ambition" [1]

Once we understand the nature of physical fitness and physical training adaptations, we must decide on the type of exercise we will use (mode), how much time we have to spend in an activity (duration), and how much effort we are able to devote to attaining fitness. Finally, we need to determine how often (frequency) and how hard (intensity) we can pursue our goals. If we decide organized games, sports, or exercising will be the method that we want to use and feel that we are not particularly experienced with these activities, we should join some group or organization like a health club, YMCA, or some type of school program where there is supervision and experienced staff.

PHYSICAL ACTIVITY AND EXERCISE APPROACHES
"Doing is activity; and he will still be doing." [2]

There are three general approaches to physical activity. These approaches include a purposeful physically active lifestyle; secondly, competitive athletics, as well as recreational sports and games; and thirdly, physical exercise, calisthenics, and work-out activities. Each of these approaches has its own unique benefit and if they are performed collectively and regularly they will contribute to the maintenance and improvement of physical fitness. **"Wise men say it is the wisest course."[3]** It is well established that physical activity can facilitate good health, enhance energy levels, and delay many of the effects of aging. Further, the benefits of physical activity not only extend into the areas of physical health and well being, but also improved emotional and psychological well-being.

---

1   Hamlet, Act II Sc. II
2   King Henry V, Act III, Sc. VII
3   King Henry VI, part III, Act III, Sc. I

> "There is a tide in the affairs of men,
> Which, taken at the flood, leads on to fortune;
> Omitted, all the voyage of their life
> Is bound in shallows and in miseries." [4]

Purposeful Physically Active Lifestyles

> "The labour we delight in physics pain." [5]

Purposeful physical activity is not necessarily planned and structured, not easily quantified, measured or timed. It is what our ancestors had to do, and what people today should *try* to do as we get through our daily lives. Today, more than any other time in history, people's daily work or employment lacks, if not totally discourages opportunities for physical activity. **"Doing the execution and the act"** [6] is a concept that should become an integral part of our daily lives. Like bathing, combing hair or brushing teeth, we should attempt to include physical activity in our work and daily lives wherever and whenever possible.

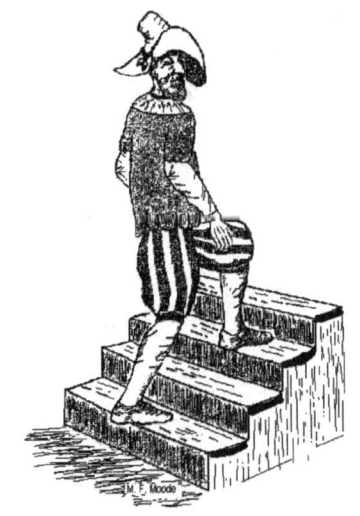

> **"I have of late-but wherefore I know not—
> lost all my mirth,
> forgone all custom of exercises; and indeed
> it goes so heavily
> with my disposition ... "** [7]

Instead of reserving our exercise to the athletic courts, fields, weight rooms or gymnasiums we should change our lifestyles to include more physical activity by deliberately, constantly, and emphatically changing our usual behaviors. Take the stairs whenever possible. Drive less. If we must drive we should park a few blocks away, or at least at the far end of a parking lot and walk to our destination. Or, perhaps we could drive our personal cars as if they were rental cars with mileage charges. We might set conservative mileage limits for ourselves and every mile we exceed the limit per day, or week, or month we should pay to a special account twenty-five cents for each mile over our limit. This approach may well make us more conscious of how much, or how often we ride or

---

4   Julius Caesar, Act IV, Sc. III
5   Macbeth, Act II, Sc. III
6   King Henry V, Act II, Sc. II
7   Hamlet, Act II, Sc. II

drive. In the worst case scenario it could contribute to a formidable medical account to help us through our deteriorating, declining physical lives!

"When thou didst ride in triumph through the streets." 8

We should consider walking or cycling to work. If we use public transportation, consider getting off a few blocks before or after our stop and do a little extra walking. In our daily work we must consciously try to include physical activity. Minimize phone conversations that could be done in person. Deliver notes, forms and reports in person rather than by inter-office mail, e-mail, FAX or telephone. During our sedentary work-days we should perform stretches and walk around. We should never use elevators or escalators. We should take a brisk walk when we get the urge to snack. At home we should do our own yard work. Mowing with a push mower is an excellent form of physical activity. Walking to the market, carrying our own groceries instead of using a shopping cart and walking home likewise could be excellent practical activities.

"I am a true labourer: I earn that I eat" 9

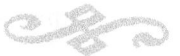

SPORTS AND GAMES

"the purpose of playing, whose end, both at the first and now, was and is, to hold, as 'twere, the mirror up to nature" 10

Physical activity that involves sports and games is a common part of virtually all advanced societies. We are blessed with all manner of labor saving devices and leisure time and in spite of this good fortune we still possess the physiological need for physical activity. It is a tragic yet common preference but most modern societies have chosen to meet their activity needs and fill their incredible amounts of free time by "hanging-out," being "cool," and occasionally engaging in sports and games. These behaviors are common among the young. As we mature, we become increasingly more sedentary and dedicated to *watching* sports and activities.

"his addiction was to courses vain, His companies unletter'd, rude and shallow, His hours fill'd up with riots, banquets, sports" 11

Athletic and recreational sports and games often demand explosive bursts of physical effort from participants. Additionally, sports and games are competitive in nature, measured,

---

8 King Henry VI, part II, Act II, Sv IV
9 As You Like It, Act III, Sc. II
10 Hamlet, Act III, Sc. II
11 King Henry V, Act I, Sc. I

scored, and usually timed with a clear and distinct beginning and a definite completion or end. A major draw back with sports and games is that they often include regular rest periods and breaks and therefore contribute only minimally to the components of physical fitness. Additionally, participation is usually on an irregular basis except for professional athletes or young intercollegiate or interscholastic athletes who practice regularly and condition themselves continuously and systematically.

"better to be eaten to death with a rust than to be scoured to nothing with perpetual motion." [12]

Another problem and common misconception is the deep-seated and widely held belief that youthful sport participation or professional sports will serve the athlete for his or her entire lifetime. This is a spectacular fallacy! Sport fitness is sport fitness and physical fitness is physical fitness and though they can and sometimes do overlap they are not necessarily the same thing! Intense sport training and therefore sport fitness can span an athlete's mid-teen years through perhaps the late twenties to mid thirties. Following this time, an athlete's best performing, competing, and training days are over and with the end of sport training sport fitness levels begin to diminish. **"Youth is full of sport, age's breath is short." [13]**

There is an indirect benefit to sport training that is often overlooked and has little to do with sport itself. Those who engage in sport and regular training learn their physical limits and become comfortable with their body's ability to endure physical distress and activity pain. **"My duty then shall pay me for my pains." [14]** The person who has never experienced *sport training* probably has never tested the limits of physical performance. This being the case, when out of necessity or choice a person tries to gain or improve physical fitness they might misinterpret and overreact to the discomfort and unfamiliar pain that can result from physical activity. Misunderstanding these new and unusual aches and pains makes quitting the pursuit of physical fitness more likely.

Physical fitness, whether for sports or for our daily lives is like electricity—it is generated, utilized, and consumed at the instant that it is needed. When athletes cease their training or we non-athletes settle in to our sedentary lifestyles the fitness we may have possessed begins to diminish and disappear. Fitness, whether sport or physical, cannot be *stored*, *saved*, or *stashed away* for use later in life.

**"For violent fires soon burn out themselves;
Small showers last long, but sudden storms are short" [15]**

12	King Henry VI, part II, Act I, Sc. II
13	Sonnet XII.
14	All's Well that Ends Well, Act II, Sc. I
15	King Richard II, Act II, Sc. I

Dreams Are Indeed Ambition

In contrast to athletes, most of us engage in sports sporadically conditioning our physical selves erratically if at all.

"Thy exercise hath been too violent" [16]

With this inconsistent and irregular approach to sports and games, rather than contributing to positive and improved fitness adaptations, the physical activity is just as likely to put us at increased risk of **"anguish, pain and agony."**[17] **"There be some sports are painful."**[18] These difficulties result from a lack of appropriate conditioning and an inability to adapt to activity.

"it is virtuous to be constant in any undertaking." [19]

Exercise, Calisthenics, and Work-Out Activities

" ... allow me such exercises as may become a gentleman" [20]

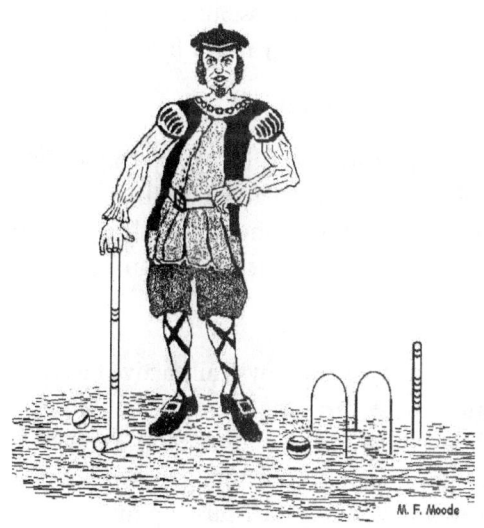

Exercise is physical activity for its own sake—planned, structured, and often performed repetitively. Exercises that require total-body involvement can contribute to the maintenance, of or may even improve, physical fitness. Exercise programs include calisthenics, yoga, stretching, weight or resistance activities, various types of rhythmic step exercises, as well as walking, jogging, running, cycling, and swimming. Organized programs through health clubs, schools, gymnasiums, parks, and recreation fitness centers, **"the common show-place, where they exercise"** [21] are easy to find and are usually professionally supervised.

16	Coriolanus, Act I, Sc. V
17	King Richard III, Act IV, Sc. IV
18	The Tempest, Act III, Sc. I
19	Measure for Measure, Act III, Sc. II
20	As You Like It, Act I, Sc. I
21	Antony and Cleopatra, Act III, Sc. VI

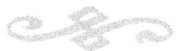

The Value of a Physically Active Lifestyle

"The elements be kind to thee, and make Thy spirits all of comfort!" [22]

The preceding modes of physical activity are effective stressors that are capable of leading to physical fitness.

"The rich advantage of good exercise." [23]

One weakness that should be remembered is that virtually all of these activities, except for purposeful work, are for lack of a better description—*contrived*. This does not diminish their potential for contributing to and resulting in training adaptations. However, they are not necessarily natural or a common part of most people's lives. They are auxiliary physical activities that we engage in to compensate for our generally motionless, minimally-active lives. To attain true physical fitness, physical activity should be a regular part of everyone's life. Instead of living our lives around specific hours of activity or scheduled exercise sessions we should try to permanently change our *lifestyles* by incorporating more physical activity in our lives *everyday*.

"The noble change that I have purposed" [24]

It is important to remember that muscles used in any activity, any time of day, can and do contribute to physical fitness. Walking as a means of transportation, carrying, lifting, moving around should be a regular and customary part of everyone's life. Then the previously discussed *contrived* activities become truly valuable as supplemental forms of activity, contributing to even higher levels of fitness as well as health and wellness.

Today, most people recognize and believe that sports, exercise and physically active lifestyles will improve or maintain the function and condition of the various components of physical fitness. **"For any or for all these exercises"** [25] can, under some circumstances, contribute to health, may help maintain fitness and improved physiological function. However, in our car-driving, trash-compacting, computer-game-playing, shopping-cart-pushing lives we not only avoid purposeful physical activity, we evade and shun activity at every opportunity.

"He is of late retired from court And is less frequent to his princely exercises Than formerly he hath appeared." [26]

22	Antony and Cleopatra, Act III, Sc. II
23	King John, Act IV, Sc. II
24	King Henry IV, part II, Act IV, Sc. V
25	The Two Gentlemen of Verona, Act I, Sc. III
26	The Winters' Tale, Act Iv, Sc. II

Elevators, escalators, automatic door openers, television remote controls and absolutely no lifting, carrying or moving of any object (except food), we pass our lives **"upon a lazy bed the livelong day."** [27]

Today competitive and recreational sports, a variety of exercises, and even a deliberate physically active lifestyle are pursued and have become a part of our lives with the vague notion that ". . . . **having, and in quest to have"** [28] our health, fitness, and lives will be enhanced and improved.

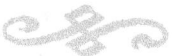

Elizabethan Activity and Lifestyles

" **... service shall with steeled sinews toil,
And labour shall refresh itself with hope ... "** [29]

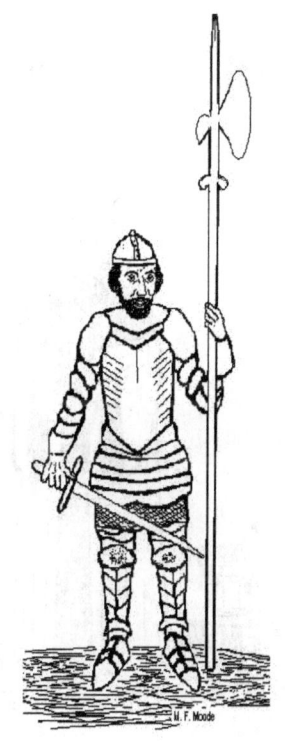

By contrast, in Elizabethan England whatever sport or competition that did exist was primarily related to military preparation and battle.

" **... they have been thoughtful to invest
Their sons with arts and martial exercises"** [30]

The concept of recreational sport was virtually non-existent in Shakespeare's time. Whatever sport and recreation there was, was the privilege of a very small leisure class - primarily the nobility and royalty. The **"princes, barons, lords, knights, squires ... gentlemen of blood and quality"** [31] were a very small and exclusive group and the only group that possessed free or spare time for recreational activity. In Elizabethan England there was very little leisure time or inclination on the part of the citizenry to engage in what we would call recreational sports or games. The concept of exercise, that is physical activity for its own sake, and for the health and fitness benefits that it would lead to, was a totally unfamiliar and unknown concept. Purposeful activity was what characterized virtually all of Elizabethan society. All aspects of life were characterized by physical exertion, effort and labor. Transportation, production, manufacture, virtually every part of daily life was based upon human toil,

---

27 Troilus and Cressida, Act I, Sc. III
28 Sonnet, CXXIX
29 King Henry V, Act II, Sc. II
30 King Henry IV, part II, Act IV, Sc. V
31 King Henry, Act IV, Sc. VIII

muscular endeavors and physical drudgery. In this type of environment, pursuit of sport, recreational competition, exercise for the sake of exercise, or physical work for any potential benefit was not even a remote consideration.

"I have no superfluous leisure" [32]

Relief from physical effort and the pursuit of comfort, recuperation, and repose were what motivated most people in Shakespeare's England.

ACTIVITY PRECAUTIONS AND PREPARATION

"Advise him to a caution" [33]

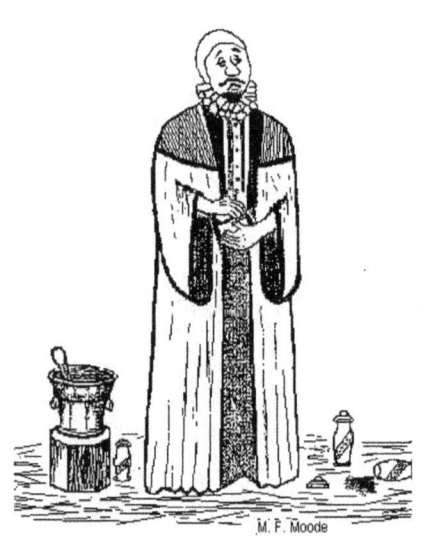

Before committing to a systematic fitness activity program or substantially increasing the activity in our normally sedentary lives, it is a good idea to undergo a medical evaluation by a physician—especially as we get older.

"Though I look old, yet I am strong and lusty" [34]

This procedure should detect any physical or health risks and is important in order to determine if increased physical activity has the potential to contribute to fitness or perhaps be dangerous and not promote fitness at all.

"bid them rise, and live" [35]

Elderly and sedentary individuals that begin an activity program after years of neglect should proceed slowly and under a doctor's supervision. This is even more important if the exercise or activity is associated with rehabilitation. If, during activity, symptoms of dizziness, nausea, excessive shortness of breath or chest pain occur, stop the activity immediately.

32	Measure For Measure, Act III, Sc. I
33	Macbeth, Act III, Sc. VI
34	As You Like It, Act II, Sc. III
35	Troilus and Cressida, Act V, Sc. III

"No longer exercise
Upon a valiant race thy harsh
And potent injuries"[36]

Once it has been determined that increased activity and regular exercise will not be detrimental, then these vigorous exercise activities should be approached in a systematic manner.

"prepare the body then"[37]

Three elements of any and all exercise programs must be determined. They are duration, frequency, and intensity. Duration or time considerations include how long and when activity should take place. Frequency considerations are related to how often activity will be engaged in, while intensity is related to how difficult or how intense the activity should be. Another general concern is a "warm-up." Stretching exercises and warm-up exercises are not necessarily the same thing and should not be confused. A warm-up or brief, comfortable cardiovascular activity should be completed before exercise. The warm-up increases blood flow throughout the body, increases the temperature of muscles, and increases the temperature of the body generally. If flexibility exercises are performed before you engage in exercise they should be preceded by warm-up activities. Warming up before performing flexibility exercises enhances range of motion of the joints, reduces the possibility of injury and soreness, and improves muscle function. Such activities as a brisk walk or comfortable jog, riding a stationary bicycle or any activity that is continuous, rhythmic, and uses large muscle groups is ideal for warm-up activities. We must be careful to perform the warm-up by starting at a slow gentle pace and gradually increasing the intensity until we approach our target-zone heart rate. This physiological warm-up will increase the temperature of the muscles, increase circulation and slightly increase body temperature. **"If you might please to stretch it."** [38] Next, stretching activities should be performed in order to prepare the muscles for the activity which is to follow. This will minimize the possibility of soft tissue injury which might result from muscles and tendons which may be unnecessarily tight and unprepared for movement.

Upon the completion of an exercise session a cool-down activity session should follow. This process usually involves continued mild exercise such as slow jogging or brisk walking. This procedure helps cool the body slowly; clears metabolic wastes from the muscles and tissues that have been recently worked; and minimizes the potential for pain and soreness which might result from the exercise that proceeded. **"Let me live, and feel no pain."**[39] It is well known and widely accepted that a cool-down phase of activity

---

36 Cymbeline, Act V, Sc. I
37 Julius Caesar, Act III, Sc.I
38 King Henry VIII, Act II, Sc. III
39 King Henry VI, part II, Act III, Sc. III

following vigorous exercise will reduce the occurrence and severity of muscle stiffness and pain that may occur during subsequent hours and days.

Duration

"I wasted time, and now doth time waste me" [40]

How much time should we devote to additional physical activity? The answer in today's **"most brisk and giddy-paced times"**[41] is often misguided and frequently wrong. Generally, a minimum of twenty to thirty continuous minutes, three days per week (with days off in between) at an intensity of sixty percent to ninety percent of maximum heart rate is the standard recommendation. Activity duration of less than thirty minutes is not necessarily a bad thing but it does not allow enough time for the body to begin to adapt positively and improve. **"So many hours must I sport myself"** [42] Recently, the view of exercise duration has changed and there are those who advocate as little as thirty minutes per day. Further, it is felt that exercise does not necessarily need to be continuous. Ten minutes here, five minutes there during a twenty-four hour period, as long as we complete thirty minutes of working-out is now viewed as a desirable minimum time commitment.

> **"Thereby to see the minutes how they run,**
> **How many make the hour full complete;**
> **How many hours bring about the day;**
> **How many days will finish up the year;**
> **How many years a mortal man may live."** [43]

However, we should ask ourselves if this mincing of minutes, the seeking of the least time commitment at the greatest convenience, actually fulfills the spirit and reflects a physically active lifestyle. We are frequently encouraged by exercise equipment manufacturers, fitness authorities, and our own inclinations to commit ourselves to the *least* amount of time. We are always willing to believe that some new exercise device, training technique, diet, or pill is the magic that will allow us to achieve maximum results with minimum time commitment. In seeking fitness gains with minimal time spent, we are in fact denying thousands of years of human existence, and survival. Effective and desirable physical fitness results cannot be achieved without reasonable and appropriate time and effort expenditures.

> **"Haste still pays haste, and leisure answers leisure;**
> **Like doth quit like, and measure still for measure."** [44]

40	King Richard II, Act V Sc. V
41	Twelfth Night, Act II, Sc. IV
42	King Henry VI, part III, Act II, Sc. V
43	King Henry VI, part III, Act II, Sc. V
44	Measure Fore Measure, Act V, Sc. I

Continuous physical activity that lasts a long time, sixty minutes or more, of moderate intensity has the greatest positive fitness benefits. Fitness programs or fitness activities of at least this duration are the most likely to result in cardiorespiratory improvement, fat loss and positive training adaptations. Conversely, exercise programs of short duration and high intensity do not necessarily contribute to or benefit physical fitness.

Generally, physical activity or exercise that can be performed continuously for a long time contributes to reduced risk of heart disease. Though many people and even some organizations work at fitness through short duration and intense physical efforts these approaches should be viewed with skepticism and caution. The attainment and maintenance of physical fitness, coupled with a nutritious diet and reasonable rest patterns, require dedication to a long-term, systematic investment in an active life.

Frequency
"Many a time and often ... " [45]

How often we are able to engage in activity is obviously and directly determined by our daily work demands, commitments to family and friends, and of course motivation. After we have decided that we are going to incorporate purposeful physical activity into our lives and decided what additional physical activities will be performed, we must determine how often we can pursue our activities in order to realize the greatest benefit. Generally, a minimum of three to four activity days per week are acceptable. However, it should be understood that a regular physically active life is best and definitely the basis upon which physical fitness should be grounded. Setting aside time to exercise every day, or every other day, for so many hours is an acceptable activity supplement but we must appreciate and understand that we cannot and should not save or hoard opportunities to be physically active. Fitness experts advise that in order to achieve optimal fitness levels, we should supplement our otherwise physically dynamic lifestyles with exercise at least three to four times a week, in an appropriate aerobic zone, for a minimum of thirty minutes.

---

45   Timon of Athens, Act III, Sc. I

Intensity

"It shall be full of poise and difficult weight" [46]

Intensity of physical activity refers to the severity or stress that an activity places on the cardiorespiratory system. Young, healthy people, or people who have maintained an active lifestyle certainly may and often do determine their own exercise intensity.

"young in limbs, in judgment old" [47]

Physical activity should be performed comfortably with no undue distress or pain. The common athletic cliché that there is no gain without pain or as Shakespeare might say **"pain purchased doth inherit pain"** [48] is not only unsound, it may be dangerous.

"My legs can keep no pace with my desires. Here will I rest me till the break of day" [49]

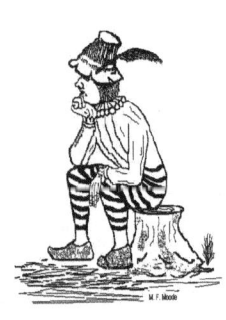

Subjective feelings of comfort or pain are not good indicators of activity intensity. The best and certainly easiest way to judge exercise intensity is to keep track of your heart rate during activity. This is accomplished by counting your pulse beats. The procedure for doing this is simple. Immediately after activity or exercise but definitely within five seconds of quitting, count your own pulse beats at your neck or wrist for ten seconds. Pulse rate decreases rapidly after exercise ceases so you must begin counting immediately. Multiply the pulse beats you counted for ten seconds by six to convert the beats you counted into beats per minute. When at rest the heart rate, therefore the pulse, is typically about seventy-two beats per minute. When a person engages in sport, physical exercise, or any kind of physical activity, the heart rate (pulse) increases in direct response to the intensity of the activity.

"A merry heart goes all the day" [50]

There is a threshold heart rate above which you should raise your pulse in order to achieve a positive training effect. Once the threshold is exceeded it is desirable that we maintain this higher heart rate for as long a time as possible. The threshold needed to achieve a training effect is lower for people who are very sedentary compared to the very fit. Associated with

---

46	Othello, Act III Sc. III
47	The Merchant of Venice, Act II, Sc. VII
48	Love's Labour's Lost, Act I Sc. I
49	A Midsummer Night's Dream, Act III, Sc. II
50	The Winters Tale, Act IV, Sc. III

Dreams Are Indeed Ambition

the threshold heart rate is the concept that there is a heart rate range or zone in which you should maintain your heart rate for an extended period of time (duration) in order to ensure positive physical adaptations. Engaging in activity with a heart rate that is below the lower end of the heart rate range is probably insufficiently intense to contribute to a training effect. Conversely, engaging in activity with a heart rate that is above the heart rate range **"is wasteful and ridiculous excess"** [51] and does not necessarily guarantee a training effect.

"I doubt not but thy training hath been noble" [52]

Calculating our target training heart rate range is a simple process. First we must subtract our age from the number two hundred twenty. This calculation tells us our age-adjusted maximum heart rate. The age-adjusted maximum heart rate next should be multiplied to determine the exercise heart rate range. First multiply the age adjusted maximum heart rate by .6. Next multiply the age adjusted maximum heart rate by .8. These multiplications give us the recommended upper and lower range of heart rates that we should work within if we are healthy, reasonably fit, and working on maintaining or improving physical fitness. If we are badly out of shape, new to exercise, or simply a beginner, we would use .6 and then .7 as the multiplicand numbers. If we are well conditioned and working at pushing our fitness level to its highest potential, we should use .8 and then .9 as the multiplicand numbers.

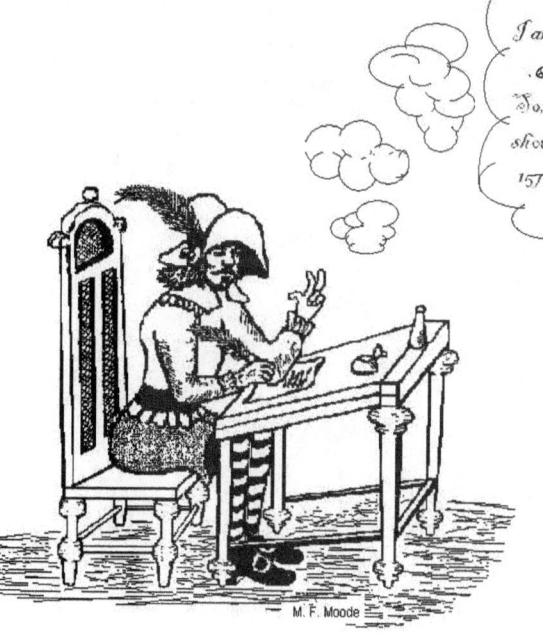

Lets see . . . .
I am 24 years old, therefore 220 - 24 = 196.
.6 X 196 = 118.   .8 X 196 = 157.
So, to achieve maximum fitness benefits I should keep my heart rate between 118 and 157 beats per minute while exercising.

Heart rate range indicates the upper and lower limits of heart rates that are sufficient to result in a physical training effect. Engaging in physical activity and maintaining the heart rate within the lower and upper range is generally an effective and efficient way to exercise and achieve the desired training effect.

---

51   King John, Act IV, Sc. II
52   Pericles, Prince of Tyre, Act IV, Sc. VI

To This Good Purpose

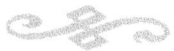

Chapter IV

Exercise Activities

**"May I never
To this good purpose, that so fairly shows,
Dream of impediment!"** [1]

Physical fitness is most easily and more likely maintained by living a life that includes regular, purposeful physical activity. **"In doing it, pays itself."** [2] Continual physically active lifestyles will contribute to fitness levels that are adequate to handle routine daily demands, foster good health and physiological function, and expend surplus energy (calories) that we in our **"luxurious, avaricious"** [3] lives often and easily consume beyond the amounts of energy we need. Physically active lifestyles can and do contribute to a long life. If we wish to achieve even greater degrees of fitness, it then becomes necessary to engage in a fitness program. The greatest challenge is not learning new skills, activities, or proper technique, how many sets or reps to do, or how much weight to lift. It is deciding how to change the sedentary routines that characterize our lives.

" ... **change misdoubt to resolution: Be that thou hopest to be** ... " [4]

Physical activity and exercise should be comfortable, convenient, and easily achieved. If you have to drive to get to a gym, weight room, or jogging track, the act of exercising may become an unpleasant task. If you spend more time traveling to the gym than you do engaging in activity, you should consider a program that is closer to home, closer to work or literally and figuratively in between the two. We must understand that there is a difference between exercise activities, **"More plentiful than tools"** [5] and exercise programs. **"Go to it orderly."** [6] Most people's fitness training involves individual activities such as walking, jogging, running, swimming or cycling. These physical efforts are useful movement activities that certainly are able to maintain or improve physical

---

1   Antony and Cleopatra, Act II, Sc. II
2   Macbeth, Act I, Sc. IV
3   Macbeth, Act IV, Sc. III
4   King Henry VI, part II, Act III, Sc. I
5   Cymbeline, Act V, Sc. III
6   The Taming of the Shrew, Act II, Sc.I

fitness. However, these exercise activities by themselves usually effect only one or two fitness components at a time. No single exercise is best or improves all components or physical fitness simultaneously. By contrast, an exercise program is a combination of training exercises which are intended to maintain or improve all fitness components during a work-out session.

"Therefore let our alliance be combined." [7]

There are many sound exercise activities to choose from in developing an exercise program. It is important to understand that the best exercise programs should consist of at least three or more exercise activities. Today jogging is widely believed to be the most fashionable, easiest, and most effective mode of exercise. It is generally held that for cardiorespiratory fitness and enhanced body composition, as well as ease of performance and convenience, jogging is the best and most effective exercise that a person may perform. The problem with emphasizing jogging, **"this false sport"** [8] or any single exercise activity, is that performing only one activity cannot and will not contribute to each of the different components of physical fitness. No one exercise activity is best for maintaining or improving all of the components of physical fitness at one time. The avid jogger should include other exercise activities as a regular part of the training program.

The exercise approach commonly referred to as cross-training has developed and become widely practiced in recent years. By performing a variety of complementary activities, by cross-training, you can work different areas of your body, different components of fitness, prevent boredom, and minimize the chance of injuries. Conversely, engaging in a single fitness activity all of the time will be less effective and quickly lead to boredom **"and thus the native hue of resolution is sicklied o'er with the pale cast of thought, and enterprises of great pith and moment with this regard their currents turn awry, and lose the name of action."** [9] Fitness activities that are **"sweetly varied"** [10] **"in different pleasures"** [11] are the most effective. When we understand the benefits that can be achieved from a wide range of physical activities then the only decision we must make is what activities we enjoy.

Flexibility Exercises

"Her blood is settled, and her joints are stiff" [12]

7	Julius Caesar, Act IV, Sc. I
8	A Midsummer Night's Dream, Act III, Sc. II
9	Hamlet, Act III, Sc. I
10	Love's Labour's Lost, Act IV, Sc. II
11	Timon of Athens, Act I, Sc. I
12	Romeo and Juliet, Act IV, Sc. V

Flexibility is the capacity to move joints through a full range of motion. It is an important and often overlooked component of physical fitness. The ability to comfortably move through a full range of motion without pain is essential to enjoy a full and complete life. In modern society we tend to become less flexible as we grow older, experience more difficulty in performing simple movements and experience more aches and pains following physical activity. **"Aches contract and starve your supple joints!"** [13] As flexibility declines, our muscles become tighter, motion is painful, and we have a hard time accomplishing everyday tasks.

"Yet all goes well, yet all our joints are whole." [14]

Simple things like getting dressed, tying our shoelaces, reaching overhead to get something off a high shelf, or getting up from a comfortable chair are often difficult with diminished or limited flexibility. When joints can move comfortably through a full range of motion it signifies more than just joint health it also indirectly signifies that bones and muscles are regularly used and are probably functioning well.

"Good arms, strong joints" [15]

A basic understanding of joint structure can contribute to and facilitate the improvement of flexibility. A joint is simply a place where two or more bones come together and are capable of moving. The bony shape and structure of joints are the primary factors that determine how much movement will be possible. Generally, ligaments like the aforementioned joint shape cannot be greatly changed to enhance joint flexibility. However, soft tissues are also important factors in limiting motion of a joint. Soft tissues include tendons, muscles and fat. Excessive amounts of fat can act like a wedge at a joint and thereby limit movement. Muscles and muscle tendons are where stretching exercises are directed and where flexibility can be maintained and improved. **"Against them both my true joints bended be."** [16] Flexibility exercises are movements and activities which are intended to improve the range of motion of a specific joint or joints. Flexibility exercises increase muscle length and thereby facilitate and enhance joint movement. Increasing muscle length is the best way to improve range of motion in normal healthy functioning joints.

"Till bones and flesh and sinews fall away" [17]

Flexibility may be developed, maintained, or even improved by using a number of exercise approaches in a gradual process. In contrast to other fitness exercise activities, flexibility exercises may be performed on a regular daily basis and are perfectly safe and beneficial. Three days per week of exercising would be considered the minimum commitment in order

---

13   Timon of Athens, Act I, Sc. I
14   King Henry IV, part I, Act IV, Sc. I
15   Troilus and Cressida, Act I, Sc. III
16   King Richard II, Act V, Sc. III
17   King Henry VI, part I, Act III, Sc. I

to maintain flexibility. As flexibility improves, it is desirable to increase the number of exercise repetitions and to increase the time that each stretch is sustained. There is evidence to suggest that maximum flexibility gains will occur when each stretch is held for at least ten seconds, thirty seconds being a maximum. To hold a stretching exercise longer is inefficient and will result in no greater improvement than a thirty-second stretch. Finally, as you hold a stretch it should become easier if we focus on muscle relaxation.

"The motion's good indeed and be it so" [18]

For the purpose of physical fitness there is one commonly used stretching approach which is safe, sound, and effective. The technique is referred to as static stretching. Static stretching involves movements performed slowly, as far as possible and to a point of mild discomfort, then holding the extreme position for the recommended ten to thirty seconds.

Performed regularly and correctly, static stretching can effectively increase muscle length and contribute to increased range of motion. Static stretch movements require that we assume a stretch position moving slowly to the extreme range of motion where muscle tightness becomes extremely uncomfortable and then hold that position. **"Of sufferance comes ease."** [19] Control must be maintained as we try to move to the extreme range of joint motion. Static flexibility exercises should go to the extreme limit of normal motion. Static stretch positions should not be forced to the extent that it causes pain.

"Extremely stretch'd and conn'd with cruel pain" [20]

The extreme position places an increased demand on the joint and muscles and results in improved muscle length and therefore enhanced joint motion. The person performing stretching exercises must try to relax the muscles being worked. With muscles relaxed, the forces creating or causing the exercise come from body weight and gravity, not from muscle action. This type of flexibility exercise can contribute significantly to fitness flexibility.

Static stretches should be a regular part of all warm-up and cool-down activities. Static stretches are safer than most other stretch techniques, they occur **"betwixt a benefit and an injury'** [21] and you are far less likely to overstretch and cause damage.

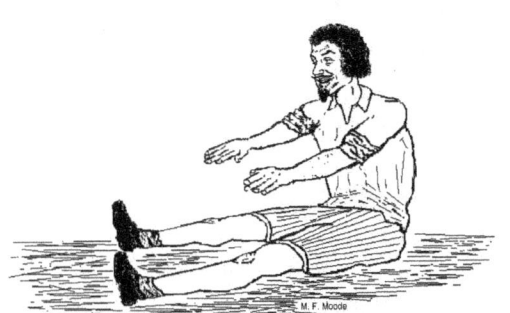

"My every action to be guided by others' experiences." [22]

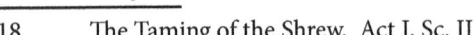

18	The Taming of the Shrew, Act I, Sc. II
19	King Henry IV, part II, Act V, Sc. IV
20	A Midsummer Night's Dream, Act V, Sc. I
21	Othello, Act I, Sc. III
22	Cymbeline, Act I, Sc. IV

In order to improve or maintain flexibility the following guidelines are suggested:

Flexibility activities should precede and follow every exercise session.
"That is the true beginning of our end." [23]

When performing flexibility activities care should taken so as not to force joints beyond their normal ranges of motion—rather exercise should be to the point of extreme discomfort not pain.
"Why force you this?" [24]

While performing flexibility activities, concentrate on relaxing the muscles which are being stretched. The more relaxed a muscle is the less likely it is to be injured during flexibility activities.
"So; now, methinks, I feel a little ease." [25]

Flexibility exercises should be performed on both sides of the body.
"On both sides more respect." [26]

Each joint flexibility exercise should be repeated four or five times during the warm-up and cool-down exercise session.
"repeat their semblance often. . . ." [27]

Because flexibility is joint specific, exercises must be performed at each joint in which flexibility development or maintenance is desired.
" ... thy charge exactly is perform'd: but there's more work." [28]

Unless stretching activities are performed through a full range of motion, the activity will probably be ineffective.
"Setting endeavour in continual motion" [29]

Another approach to flexibility are ballistic types of stretching exercises. Ballistic stretches are movements that many misinformed people utilize in order to maintain or improve their physical fitness and flexibility. These types of stretches involve bouncing or jerking movements of body parts or muscles that are being stretched. This type of movement may contribute to some sport movements and performance skills but seldom has a positive effect on physical fitness. Generally, ballistic stretching is not considered sound and can lead to injury.

---

23   A Midsummer Night's Dream, Act V, Sc. I
24   Coriolanus, Act II, Sc. II
25   King Henry VIII, Act IV, Sc. II
26   Coriolanus, Act III, Sc. I
27   King Henry VI, part I, Act V, Sc. III
28   The Tempest, Act I, Sc. II
29   King Henry, Act I, Sc. II

"like an engine, wrench'd my frame" [30]

Ballistic movements do not allow muscles to adapt to, or relax in the stretched position and may, instead result in or cause tighter shortened muscles by repeatedly activating the muscle stretch reflex. These types of flexibility activities are not necessarily suitable for or contribute to physical fitness.

Some competitive and sport activities are capable of contributing to joint flexibility improvement. Among these are some forms of dance, gymnastics, swimming and even walking. Other activities such as aerobics, running and weight lifting may also provide some benefits. Most sports activities contribute little toward improving flexibility which means that if we engage in sports, we should begin a supplemental program of systematic stretching exercises.

Muscle Properties

"Our strength is all gone into heaviness" [31]

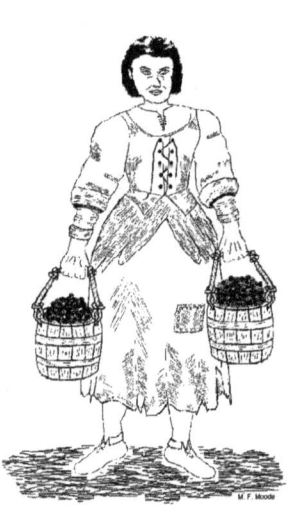

In Elizabethan times, muscle strength and endurance were essential in order to function and survive. People with suitable levels of muscle strength and endurance were able to live, work, achieve efficient movement, and therefore **"nature's fragile vessel doth sustain."** [32] Additionally, human survival was such an incredible physical struggle that just staying alive was a significant factor toward the development, maintenance, and improvement of muscle strength and endurance. In its simplest sense, muscular strength is the ability of a muscle to generate a great deal of force in a single effort.

"Some glory ... in their bodies' force ... " [33]

Force is produced by converting chemical fuels into mechanical energy which shortens muscles and moves bones. Muscular endurance is the ability of a muscle to sustain or repeat forceful exertions over a period of time.

30	King Lear, Act I, Sc. IV
31	Antony and Cleopatra, Act IV, Sc. XV
32	Timon of Athens, Act V, Sc. I
33	Sonnet XCI

"Your need to sustain" [34]

Endurance depends on the ability of muscles to produce chemical energy, and the efficient functioning of the circulatory system to transport this chemical energy and eliminate waste. Appropriate levels of muscular strength and muscular endurance are essential for good posture, for effective physiological function, and for dealing with everyday tasks. The person with adequate levels of muscle strength and endurance should experience less fatigue while working, playing, or exercising. *Power* is a property of muscles closely associated with strength. It is the ability of a muscle to generate force quickly and is essential to modern sport and competitive athletic participation. Power, in Elizabethan times, was not a particularly important aspect of a person's musculature. In our modern, sport-obsessed society, power is greatly esteemed and highly regarded.

". . . . such force and blessed power" [35]

The development of strength and endurance through various types of exercise programs and routines has become a mainstay of exercise and fitness programs in modern society.

"Let grow thy sinews till their knots be strong" [36]

When engaging in muscle exercises to improve strength or endurance, the first thing to consider is the convenience and practicality of the exercises. In **"these curious days"**[37] there is a vague notion that exercising is best and most effective if it takes place in some sort of *sacred* location like a gym, health club or exercise spa. That is, **"a place of potency and sway."** [38] This concept is not only untrue, it is often inconvenient and expensive. Muscle exercises should be convenient and the important thing is that the muscles are worked purposefully and systematically. The types of resistance used in muscle exercises can be from body weight, resistive elastic or hydraulic devices, free weights, weight machines, or any combination of the above. The key concern to sound muscle training lies in the correct exercise approach which is *progressive resistance exercise*. This approach incorporates the use of repetitive movements that result in a smooth, continuous motion. Additionally, "reps" or repetitions are grouped into sets which are a predetermined number of repetitions. Typically, an exercise will involve two or three sets of a movement that consists of ten to fifteen repetitions. Normally, after a set is completed, a rest interval follows before another set is performed by the same muscle group, or before a set for another muscle group is begun. Progressive resistance training is based on the assumption that when using substantial **"warlike resistance"** [39] or weights to train muscles, increasing resistance by increasing weight will result in enhanced strength adaptations. In a similar manner

---

34   Twelfth Night, Act IV, Sc. II
35   A Midsummer Night's Dream, Act IV, Sc. I
36   Troilus and Cressida, Act V, Sc. III
37   Sonnet XXXVIII
38   Coriolanus, Act II, Sc. III
39   All's Well That Ends Well, Act I, Sc. I

"to tire in repetition" [40] or exercise repetitions using lighter resistance will result in improved muscle endurance adaptations.

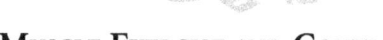

Muscle Exercise and Contractions

Isometric Exercise

"strength match'd with strength" [41]

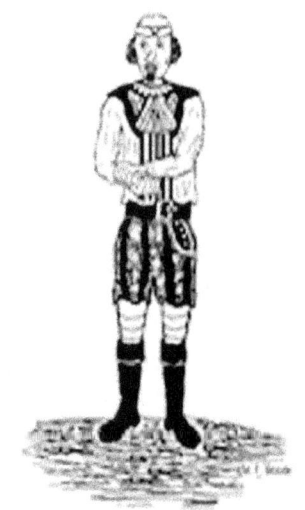

Isometrics or isometric muscle contractions are muscular exertions where force is generated but muscle length remains unchanged and there is no joint motion. These types of contractions are performed against an immovable resistance, or against an oppositional body part, such as hand against hand.

"Both are alike; and both alike we like" [42]

These types of muscle contractions and exercises are frequently used for rehabilitation since the exact area of muscle weakness can be isolated and strengthening can be administered at the appropriate joint angle. This type of exercise is easy, quick, and beneficial. It conveniently overloads and strengthens muscles without special equipment and with little chance of injury. **"Yet I alone, alone do me oppose."** [43] Isometric exercises are effective for developing strength of a particular muscle or group of muscles. However, the strength that results occurs only at the angle that the joint is exercised. This fact limits the value of isometric exercises for sport training as well as for physical fitness. One additional consideration with regard to this type of exercise is that it can contribute to increased blood pressure. The fact that the muscles are contracting with no resulting movements occludes circulation and can promote increased blood pressure.

Isotonic Exercise

"feeble force will yield at length" [44]

Isotonic muscle contractions or exercise differs from isometric exercise in that the muscles' length changes and there is joint movement during the muscle exertion.

40	Coriolanus, Act I, Sc. I
41	King John, Act II, Sc. I
42	King John, Act II, Sc. I
43	King John, Act III, Sc. I
44	Poem XIX

"is't too short? I'll lengthen it" [45]

The most common types of isotonic exercises include training with free weights, dumbbells and barbells as well as with some Universal and Nautilus type weight machines. As weights are lifted and then lowered throughout a range of motion, muscles are shortened and then lengthened. These movements, depending on the amount of weight and the number of repetitions, may contribute to strength, endurance or both depending how the exercise is performed. Muscle power may also be improved if quickness or speed is emphasized as a part of the exercise. In some exercise routines, all of the components may be improved but not necessarily equally or at the same time. When performing isotonic exercises, you **"are well foretold that danger lurks within"**[46] particularly with free weights. This because the weights being moved also need to be controlled—a circumstance which is not present with weight machines. Additionally, because of the mechanical factors of momentum and inertia associated with weights, it sometimes happens that isotonic exercises are less effective and less efficient than other forms of muscle exercises. Finally, there are exercises and various forms of calisthenics that may also be considered as a form of isotonic exercise. Activities such as chin-ups, push-ups, and sit-ups, which use body weight as the resistance force fall into this category.

ISOKINETIC EXERCISE

"How quickly should you speed?" [47]

Isokinetic muscle contractions or exercises utilize machines that control the speed of contraction through the exercise range of motion. This minimizes the momentum and inertia weakness of isotonic type contractions. **"It shall be speeded well."** [48] Isokinetic exercises combine the best features of both isometrics and isotonic weight training. It provides muscular overload at a constant preset speed while the muscle exerts force through a full range of motion.

"Constant in a wondrous excellence." [49]

Often isokinetic exercise devices get their resistance from friction, springs or hydraulic means thus requiring less control and are safer to use. For example, an isokinetic stationary bicycle set at ninety revolutions per minute means that despite how hard and fast the exerciser works, the isokinetic properties of the bike will allow the exerciser to pedal only at ninety revolutions per minute. Machines known as Cybex and Biodex provide isokinetic results; they are generally used by athletic trainers, and are not readily available to the individuals simply trying to become more physically fit.

---

45   King Henry VI, part II, Act I, Sc. II
46   King Henry VI, part III, Act IV, Sc. VII
47   Othello, Act IV, Sc. I
48   Measure for Measure, Act IV, Sc. V
49   Sonnet CV

Arise Forth from the Couch: A Shakespearean Guide to Physical Fitness

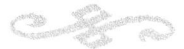

Exercising for Muscular Strength

Muscle tissue must be worked by exercise and activities that subject them to stresses beyond their **"accustomed action"** [50] to a degree of exertion which they normally do not experience. This is how the overload principle is applied to muscle strength improvement. The *overload principle*, requires that resistance be progressively increased so that the muscles are forced to work harder. When this occurs continuously, over time, and through a complete range of motion, the body will adapt specifically to the increased demands, and the ability to exert greater force will result. Strengthening exercises must be performed at the upper range of effort in the overload zone in order for muscle strength to be improved. That is at least sixty percent of the maximum strength of the muscles must be worked. **"With ... " muscles " ... encumber'd thus"**[51] to improve strength increasing the resistance rather than adding more repetitions is the best and most effective application of training specificity.

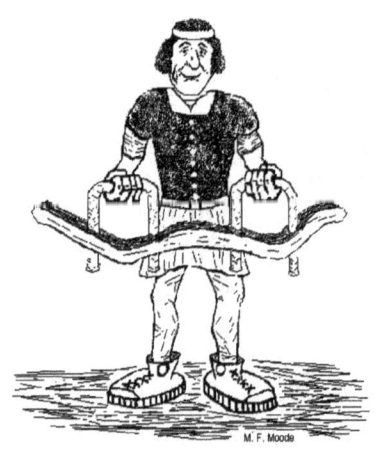

It is important to remember that muscles are arranged in opposing pairs and that as one group of muscle contracts and shortens the opposing group must relax and lengthen. **"They are opposed already."**[52] Because of this relationship it is essential to maintain a balance between opposing muscle groups and their ability to contract and shorten or stretch and lengthen. That is, as strengthening exercises are performed, in order to improve one group of muscles we must not neglect the lengthening of the opposing muscle group. **"The opposite of itself."**[53] Therefore, having strengthened and stretched appropriately we must reverse the process and strengthen and stretch in the opposite direction with the opposing muscles. These procedures will maintain joint flexibility and contribute to muscle and joint fitness. Strengthening exercises increase muscle mass, bone strength, and the body's metabolism. It can help us achieve or maintain proper weight and improve body image and self-esteem. A certain level of muscle strength is needed to perform daily activities, such as walking,

---

50   Macbeth, Act V, Sc. I
51   Hamlet, Act I, Sc. V
52   Troilus and Cressida, Act IV, Sc. V
53   Antony and Cleopatra, Act I, Sc. III

carrying objects and climbing stairs. Strengthening exercises increase muscle force by subjecting muscles to greater stresses than they normally receive. This increased stress stimulates the growth of the protein filaments inside the muscle cells that are the sites of muscle contractions. Among individuals who **"with ample and brim fulness of ... force"** [54] regularly engage in fitness activities, there are indications that strength training contributes more positively than any other type of fitness activity to self-esteem and body image. These types of benefits as well as strength improvements may all be accomplished through either isometric, isotonic or isokinetic exercises.

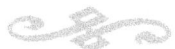

Exercising for Muscle Endurance

"to tire in repetition" [55]

Muscle endurance, like muscle strength, is improved by applying the overload and specificity principles. The overload principle emphasis should be on repetition and repeated exertions rather than maximum force.

"repeat your will and take it." [56]

A high number of repetitions, not **"too tedious to repeat"** [57] against relatively light or submaximal resistance, overloads the muscles beyond their normal comfortable working zone in such a specific way that improvement of muscle endurance results. This improvement will be specifically in the muscles worked and within the range of movement used. Generally, from the standpoint of efficiency, strength and endurance can be improved by thoughtfully and efficiently working both components within the same work-out.

Following are muscle exercise suggestions that will enhance the likelihood that strength and endurance exercises will be safe, beneficial, and successful:

Do not engage in weight lifting exercises without a spotter or attendant present. There is an element of risk when weightlifting and these types of exercises should always be performed with others around, if not involved as spotters.

"Without thy help by me be borne alone." [58]

54	King Henry V, Act I, Sc. II
55	Coriolanus, Act I, Sc. I
56	King Henry VIII, Act I, Sc. II
57	Pericles, Prince of Tyre, Act V, Sc. I
58	Sonnet XXXVI

Weight training sessions should be performed at least three times per week. Every other day is a sound approach.
"tis a chronicle of day by day"[59]

Strengthening weight exercises should be approached in a balanced way, that is we should work one muscle group and then work its opposite.
"I have in equal balance justly weigh'd" [60]

Proper breathing when weight lifting requires that you "blow the weight up **"blow them, higher and higher,"** [61] that is exhale while exerting.
"give breathing to my purpose" [62]

Stop lifting if you experience unusual discomfort or pain.
"Courage, man; the hurt cannot be much." [63]

Perform stretching exercises following all weightlifting exercise sessions.
"Give place to flexure and low bending" [64]

Walking

"sometimes he walks four hours together" [65]

Walking, which should be everyone's principal means and first choice of transportation, is also an excellent physical activity for fitness. It does not matter how fit you are, your exercise experience, body build, energy level or age—walking is an excellent activity for a lifetime. It can be performed everyday and almost anywhere. Walking is inexpensive, relatively low risk in terms of injury, and can be performed with no special equipment or athletic ability. **"We'll walk afoot awhile, and ease our legs."** [66] If fitness is the ability to respond and adapt favorably to physical activity then walking is an activity that we should be subjecting ourselves to at every opportunity! Two other positive aspects of walking are that walking can be as vigorous an activity as you want it to be and walking is capable of contributing significantly to fitness improvements.

59	The Tempest, Act V, Sc. I
60	King Henry IV, part II, Act IV, Sc. I
61	Merry Wives of Windsor, Act V, Sc. V
62	Antony And Cleopatra, Act I, Sc. III
63	Romeo and Juliet, Act III, Sc. I
64	King Henry IV, part I, Act II, Sc. I
65	Hamlet, Act II, Sc. II
66	King Henry IV, part I, Act II, Sc. II

"walking and other actual performances" [67]

It is generally recommended that thirty minutes a day is the minimum time in order to gain a training benefit from walking. Walking is an activity that virtually everyone can do and thirty minutes of walking each day likewise is not a great challenge for most people. If **"you have scarce time"** [68] for pursuing a continuous walking routine in your daily schedule, do not despair. It has been determined that shorter bouts of walking throughout the day which total thirty minutes will suffice. If you have the time and the motivation, exercise authorities have concluded that walking at a moderate pace for about an hour a day, everyday, has a substantial beneficial effect on the circulatory system, respiratory system, skeletal system, metabolism, as well as body composition.

"I have known when he would have walked ten mile a-foot" [69]

Another benefit of walking as exercise is an approach to quantifying the amount of work accomplished while walking. Fitness authorities recommend the completion of 10,000 steps every day.

"we have measured many miles." [70]

These steps need not be accomplished all in one effort or at one time. The steps may be spread out over the entire day. To facilitate the counting of our steps there are a number of devices, pedometers, that facilitate the counting of one's steps. The interesting aspect to this approach is that ten thousand does not sound as formidable or overwhelming as its equivalent distance in miles which is approximately five miles. Generally, people today average about twenty-five hundred steps or two and one half miles in their daily routine. When you walk you burn calories. The more vigorous the walk, the more calories you expend. The energy, or calories that we wish to burn, are the calories that are stored in our body's fat cells.

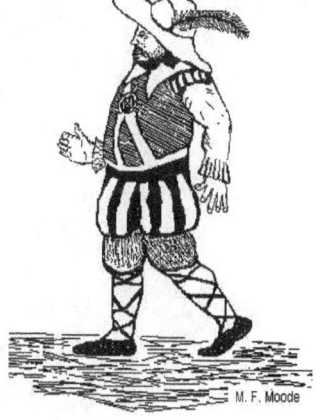
M. F. Moode

"Zounds, ye fat paunch" [71]

Walking is an activity that we can easily perform and can continue for long periods of time. Long duration activity is one of the keys to make **"less thy body hence, and more thy grace."** [72] Walking is an activity that we can undertake sometimes slowly and comfortably, sometimes

67	Hamlet, Act II, Sc. II
68	King Henry VIII, Act III, Sc. II
69	Much Ado About Nothing, Act II, Sc. III
70	Love's Labour's Lost, Act V, Sc. II
71	King Henry IV, part I, Act II, Sc. IV
72	King Henry IV, part II, Act V, Sc. V

vigorously and quickly. If we wish to lose body fat, walking is the answer. The human body will seek and utilize stored body fat as a source of energy in any activity that is performed at a moderate intensity for an long period of time. If you engage in regular walking without any reduction in dietary intake you may lose as much as a pound or two per month. While maintaining an active walking routine and reducing your caloric intake slightly, the prospect of weight loss is even better and losses even greater. Walking perhaps more than any other activity is effective, positive and safe and contributes well to improvement of all fitness components.

Jogging

"Jog on, jog on" [73]

Jogging is a popular way to exercise. Jogging is an activity that overloads and creates demands on the body's anatomical, structural, and physiological systems and thus has the potential to contribute greatly to improved physical fitness. **"You may be jogging whiles your boots are green"** [74] In reality, walking, jogging and running are all very similar. Jogging is sometimes considered a fast walk or a slow run. Jogging is similar to walking in terms of speed, but mechanically it is inherently inefficient because of its wasted vertical motions, short choppy steps that overload and contribute to its anatomical and physiological benefits.

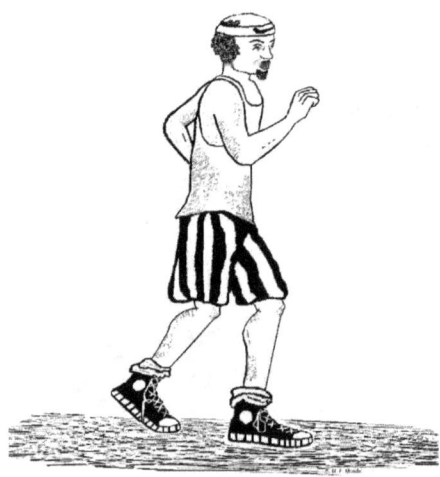

"the feet were lame and could not bear"[75]

Jogging is not without its negative aspects. Anyone who jogs needs to be aware and pay attention to how their body feels before and after jogging. The mechanical inefficiency of jogging contributes directly to all sorts of aches and pains. However, sharp pain that lasts longer than twenty to thirty minutes after a jogging session is not normal. It is important to **"know yourself"**[76] so you are alert to a muscle pull or type of injury pain that could be an indication of a more serious problem. If you experience sudden pain or serious discomfort as a result of jogging you should cease immediately

---

73   The Winter's Tale, Act IV, Sc. III
74   The Taming of the Shrew, Act III, Sc. II
75   As You Like It, Act III, Sc. II
76   As You Like It, Act III, Sc. V

and take time off until the discomfort has completely disappeared.

"readiness is all"[77]

To minimize the possibility of pain or injury when engaged in jogging you should precede and follow the jog with certain procedures. Warming up your muscles before you jog or do any exercise will minimize the risk of injury. Spend at least five to ten minutes stretching and loosening the muscles. The increased blood flow of such a warm-up will diminish any muscle tension, enhance flexibility and may improve performance and make the whole experience more pleasurable. While jogging, appropriate intensity can be easily appraised by trying to carry on a conversation. **"Conversation, that he dares in this manner assay me."** [78] Or, if jogging alone, to be able to whistle. **"Whistle blow, till thou burst thy wind."** [79] If your jogging effort is too intense you will not be able to supply enough oxygen to the working muscles and at the same time have sufficient air available for talking or whistling. If you are too out of breath to talk, you should slow down or even walk until you have recovered—then resume at your previous pace. After completing a bout of jogging, 'cool-down' by gradually reducing your jogging speed and finish your activity with a brisk walk until your heart rate and breathing return to roughly your resting rate. Finally, while your muscles are still warm from jogging, it is an ideal time to stretch and maintain or even improve muscle length and joint flexibility. As with walking for activity and exercise, long duration is far more valuable and beneficial than intensity or speed.

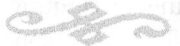

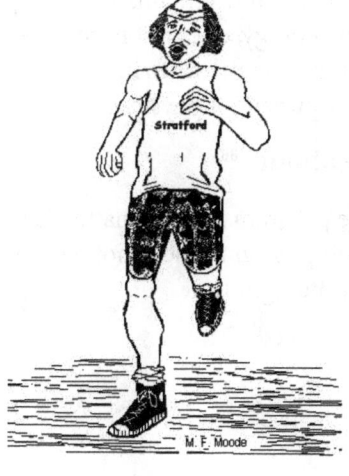

Running

"As from a bear a man would run for life" [80]

Walking, jogging, and running are all related in that they are locomotor activities and depend primarily on the legs while simultaneously alternating oppositional movements of the arms. Walking, jogging, and running are all fundamental skills and can be, performed for extended periods of time. Additionally, all of these activities are natural basic movements. Individually, they also differ from each other in their purposes, efficiency and timing. Running is rarely, if ever, appropriate for or utilized as a means of transportation. Perhaps the mechanical factor that most distinguishes running from

---

77 Hamlet, Act V, Sc. II
78 Merry Wives of Windsor, Act II, Sc. I
79 The Tempest, Act I, Sc. I
80 The Comedy of Errors, Act III, Sc. II

walking is that with running there is a period where the runner is airborne. When walking, one foot is always in contact with the ground. **"As surely as your feet hit the ground they step on."**[81] Obviously, they also differ in their speed. That is, walking is performed at a slow pace—usually around two miles per hour or less. Running usually occurs at approximately seven miles per hour or faster,—**"it requires swift foot."** [82] Jogging is usually performed **"of place 'tween high and low"** [83] between fast walking and slow running—approximately three and a half to six miles per hour. Running can be one of the most effective physical activities you can perform. Running is a fine activity for those individuals who are healthy and fit. That is, individuals with no joint or skeletal anomalies, no cardiorespiratory problems, and with normal body fat are most likely to benefit from a running program.

"Taste your legs, sir; put them to motion" [84]

Like any activity or exercise, running may not be for everyone. If it is not enjoyable, if it is unpleasant or uncomfortable it is not required! If we do enjoy running and want to include it in our exercise program, then we must take our time, progress slowly and allow bones, joints, and muscles to adapt to the physiological demands of running. **"I conjure thee but slowly; run more fast."** [85] As work-out effort progresses and we attempt to intensify our activity from walking, to jogging, to running, the body will progressively shift through and utilize each of the various means of producing energy. This shift from primarily aerobic to anaerobic energy supply will coincide with increased activity intensity that is walking, jogging, or running speed. This type of work-out progression should not necessarily be the goal of our personal physical fitness programs. Training, which continues over time and becomes progressively more severe, that reaches and remains extremely intense and relies primarily on anaerobic means of providing energy, does not necessarily enhance physical fitness. Further, this approach to physical fitness may lead to injury, pain, physical discomfort, and discourages us from continuing our pursuit of physical fitness.

"Why dost thou run so many mile about" [86]

The quickest way to end a running program, or any exercise program for that matter, is to do too much too soon. Beginning and sticking with a running program does not have to be difficult. It is simply a matter of doing the right things at the right time.

"With a good leg and a good foot" [87]

81		Twelfth Night, Act III, Sc, IV
82		Timon of Athens, Act V, Sc. I
83		Cymbeline, Act IV, Sc. II
84		Twelfth Night, Act III, Sc. I
85		King John, Act IV, Sc. II
86		King Richard III Act IV, Sc. IV
87		Much Ado About Nothing, Act II, Sc. I

To This Good Purpose

As is the case with any activity, there are procedures and techniques which should be observed if the activity is to be successful and beneficial. These techniques become even more important and critical in activities like running which involve and require high amounts of force. Following are running performance tips that **"with good advice and little medicine"**[88] will enhance the likelihood that running will be beneficial and successful:

Your head should be up and eyes forward.
"dizzy 'tis, to cast one's eyes so low!" [89]

Avoid any and all unnecessary motion and especially motion up and down.
"Have you any levers to lift me up again, being down?" [90]

If there is any body lean it should be from the ankles, not the waist.
"And gave him graceful posture." [91]

Keep your hands, arms, and shoulders relaxed, comfortable and moving only in a forward and backward direction.
"calm and gentle I proceeded" [92]

Contact the ground directly beneath your body, with your foot flat, then roll to the ball of the foot, and ultimately push off with the toes.
"My judgment is, we should not step too far"[93]

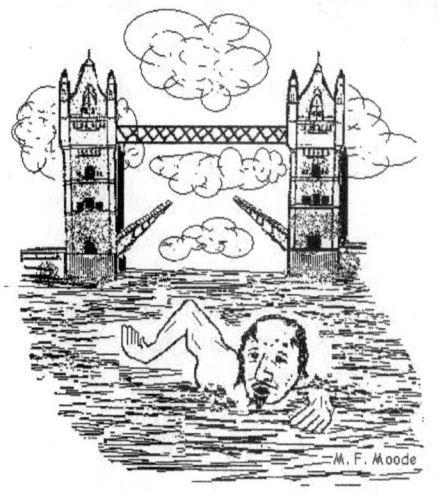

Swimming

"Leap in with me into this angry flood, And swim to yonder point" [94]

Swimming is an outstanding physical fitness activity that can be extremely vigorous or a relaxing, therapeutic, massaging alternative to other exercise activities. It is beneficial because it is very different from walking, jogging and running, and complements these activities in many positive ways. If there is a negative aspect

---

88   King Henry IV, part II, Act III, Sc. I
89   King Lear, Act IV, Sc. VI
90   King Henry IV, part I, Act II Sc. II
91   Coriolanus, Act II, Sc. I
92   Antony and Cleopatra, Act V, Sc. I
93   King Henry IV, part II, Act I, Sc. III
94   Julius Caesar, Act I, Sc. II

to swimming it is—being in the water can be an unnatural and even frightening experience. The underlying fear that is instilled in all of us from a very young age, **"sink or swim"** [95] often interferes with, and discourages **"the dauntless spirit of resolution"**[96] and we tend to live our lives avoiding aquatic activities of any kind.

"with his good arms in lusty stroke" [97]

Swimming obviously requires muscular work and therefore contributes significantly to upper-body fitness adaptations. Though walking, jogging, and running can involve the arms, shoulders, chest, and back, swimming places great demand on these body components and thereby positively works and "overloads" them more than most other fitness activities.

"careless force and forceless care" [98]

Mechanically, the pounding forces that characterize jogging and running, and to a lesser degree walking, do not occur when we exercise in water or swim. This is a mixed benefit because you sacrifice some of the bone-building adaptations of weight-bearing activities. Swimming is an excellent activity if you are recovering from an injury, such as a sprain, bruise or even some fractures. Buoyancy acts in opposition to gravity and instead of pounding the bones and joints, water floats the body, massages bones, loosens joints and contributes more significantly to the reduction of excess body fat.

" ... swim against the tide And spend her strength with over-matching waves"[99]

Caloric expenditures resulting from swimming are especially good if our fitness goal includes trying to reduce the **"portly belly,"** [100] diminish body fat, and improve body composition. Because the body experiences greater drag force and water resistance, swimming expends one-and-a-half to two times as many calories as walking, jogging or running. During the most intense efforts, swimming spends almost four times the caloric energy as fast running. A fast thirty-minute swim will consume about three hundred calories versus approximately seventy-five calories during an intense thirty-minute walk. Jogging may be easily accomplished for thirty minutes but will consume only about one hundred fifty calories. Fast running, which most of us would be hard pressed to continue for thirty-minutes, would consume approximately two hundred and twenty-five calories. Many of the calories expended during a fast run are from anaerobic sources and therefore incapable of reducing stored body fat. Additionally, fast running, except for the most highly trained individuals, would result in soreness, pain, and widespread physiological

---

95   King Henry IV, part I, Act I, Sc. III
96   King John, Act V, Sc. I
97   The Tempest, Act II, Sc. I
98   Troilus and Cressida, Act V, Sc. V
99   King Henry VI, part III, Act I, Sc. IV
100   Merry Wives of Windsor, Act I, Sc. III

upset, conditions which are rarely experienced as a result of swimming.

There are procedures and techniques which should be observed if swimming is to be pleasurable and beneficial. It is important to **"be guided by others' experiences."**[101] Following are swimming performance tips that will enhance the likelihood that swimming will be a positive fitness experience:

> The most critical factor essential to effective swimming is relaxation.
> **"methinks, I feel a little ease."** [102]

> While swimming, breathing should be rhythmic, constant, and always through the mouth.
> **"Of mortal breathing: seize it, if thou darest."** [103]

When performing a prone position stroke, the correct head position is with the head down, face in the water, and strokes should be performed rhythmically and comfortably.

> **"the elegancy, facility, and golden cadence"**[104]

Aquatic Exercise

"To melt myself away in water ... " [105]

𝔚ater exercise may be one of the best non-impact fitness activities there is and virtually anyone may take part. As is the case with swimming, the stresses and forces on weight-bearing joints, bones and muscles is reduced or non-existent when exercising in the water. **"That's a fault that water will mend"** [106] therefore, it is unlikely that a water exercise will result in injury or leave you with sore muscles. The overweight and obese, pregnant women, the elderly, people with arthritis or those recovering from an injury can all benefit from a wide variety of aquatic exercises. Additionally, the young, healthy, physically fit as well as those who are new to exercise can also benefit from water exercise.

> **"Throwing him into the water will do him a benefit"** [107]

Water exercise can work and enhance all physical fitness components. If these activities are performed regularly and for a long duration they can effectively reduce body fat. The

---

101　Cymbeline, Act I, Sc. IV
102　King Henry VII, Act IV, Sc. II
103　King Richard II, Act IV, Sc. I
104　Love's Labour's Lost, Act IV, Sc. II
105　King RIchard II, Act IV, Sc. I
106　The Comedy of Errors, Act III, Sc. II
107　Merry Wives of Windsor Act III, Sc. III

resistance of water is perfect for muscle endurance training. Instead of weights, the water itself provides the resistance. Additionally, an aquatic environment is an ideal place for performing stretches that might be difficult or impossible in a gym or exercise room. Because the effect of gravity is diminished, and balance is not a major concern, movement of the body or body parts through a wider range of motion is facilitated.

"For any or for all these exercises" [108]

An effective aquatic exercise bout should include a good warm-up. After the warm-up there should follow a work-out phase which involves cardiorespiratory and muscle endurance that gradually increase in effort **"as motion and long-during action tires"** [109] the body. Ultimately, the work-out phase slows, activity intensity diminishes until finally a "cool-down" activity phase begins. Muscle endurance can be improved easily and safely by cupping your hands and pushing or pulling the water. Other devices, such as plastic bottles filled with water, hand-held paddles, and water chutes can increase resistance to provide even more overload and a more intense work-out. Movements like running in place, stepping up and down, kicking, jumping or even dancing should be a regular part of aquatic exercise. The "cool-down" phase should include flexibility exercises for the entire body as cardiorespiratory and muscular activity is gradually diminished. Aquatic exercises are perfect for people who may find other exercises and types of movements unpleasant, too difficult, or too painful to perform on the land.

"There are no tricks in plain and simple faith" [110]

Water exercise is simple, easily performed and requires little more than a swim suit and sufficient water. Generally, there is little risk or danger involved in these activities and they can often be done individually. If however, you decide to take the plunge with other people, it is a simple matter of finding a program or class to join. Health clubs, parks and recreation pools, or community adult schools commonly offer aquatic exercise classes. It is good to visit one or two of the programs before paying money and joining to see if they are appropriate for your fitness goals. Additionally, do not hesitate to inquire about the supervisor's qualifications. Instructors should be experienced and should have certification in aquatic exercise.

---

108   The Two Gentlemen of Verona, Act I, Sc. III
109   Love's Labour's Lost, Act IV, Sc. III
110   Julius Caesar, Act IV, Sc. II

Cycling

"How many score of miles may we well ride" [111]

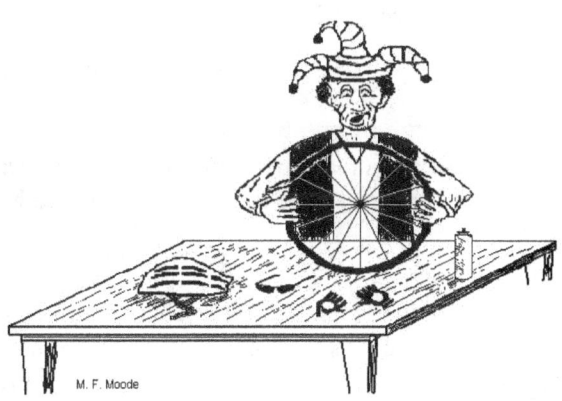

Cycling is an exceptional aerobic activity and excellent for improving cardiorespiratory endurance. It is a wonderful, cheap, and efficient means of transportation, and except for the initial day or two of bicycle seat soreness after beginning a riding program, cycling is **"all days of glory, joy and happiness."** [112] It can be enjoyed by people of all ages, requires virtually no athletic skill or ability, and beginning a riding program is easy. So easy, in fact, that a child can do it without any type of formal or complex training. In the same way as walking, jogging, running and swimming, bicycling may result in some very desirable physiological responses in terms of endurance, weight control, and overall physical fitness. Unlike many of the aforementioned fitness activities, there is virtually no evidence that bicycling is high risk or results in any overuse-type of injuries. Physicians and athletic trainers frequently prescribe indoor bicycle trainers as well as swimming, activities as a form of alternative training, therapy, and recuperation for injured athletes.

If there is a negative aspect to bicycling it is undoubtedly related to the fairly extensive assortment of equipment that is necessary **"from the crown of his head to the sole of his foot."** [113] First and foremost there is the selection, fit, purchase, and subsequently the care and maintenance of an appropriate bicycle. The main problem and perhaps biggest mistake people make when purchasing a bike is going for the image and forgetting their purpose and objectives. Racing bikes are beautiful, efficient, and sleek. Mountain bikes are rugged, strong and powerful. But if all we intend to do is ride for exercise or transportation these types of bikes are inappropriate, ineffective, and may be self defeating. Remain focused on your goals and get the right bike. The wrong bike can waste time, money, and effort and may quickly discourage us. In the same way that we would not buy a Ferrari to commute two or three miles a day, and we certainly would not buy a Mack Truck for a family vehicle, do not make these types of mistakes with your bike purchase.

---

111 Cymbeline, Act III, Sc. II
112 King John Act III, Sc. IV
113 Much Ado About Nothing, Act III, Sc. II

"go we to attire you for our journey" [114]

Next, there is a wide range of some fairly diverse and expensive equipment that facilitate safety and enhance the bicycling experience. **"Richer than wealth, prouder than garments' cost."** [115] Specially designed cycling shorts, jerseys, bicycling shoes, gloves, glasses, and various other types of gear are helpful if not essential. **"A riding-suit, no costlier than would fit."**[116] Finally, it is strongly recommended that a quality cycling helmet be purchased and worn to protect the head from injury should an accident occur.

"what quality are they of?" [117]

Bicycles come in hundreds of different styles, models, and with numerous mechanical accessories and options available. Bicycles can generally be grouped into three price ranges that roughly correspond to three different quality classifications.

"How little is the cost. . . ." [118]

A simple department store bicycle of minimal quality is usually priced slightly above a hundred dollars. At the top end of the minimally priced bicycles is the basic bicycle shop bike which usually costs about three hundred and fifty dollars. These lower end bicycles are suitable for basic transportation, light touring and exercising.

"Spare not for the cost." [119]

Mid-range bicycles cost anywhere from a minimum of three hundred and fifty dollars to seven or eight hundred dollars.

"We can afford no more at such a price." [120]

At the upper end, there are bicycles that range from eight hundred dollars up to several thousand dollars for professional touring or racing. Generally, whatever the quality you choose to ride, purchasing your bicycle from a reputable cycling shop is recommended. Bicycle shops can make sure you have the correct bicycle for you, they will make sure the bike fits properly, is correctly adjusted, appropriately tuned and equipment upgrades and repairs will be easily managed.

114	King Henry VI, part II Act II, Sc. IV
115	Sonnet XCI
116	Cymbeline, Act III, Sc. II
117	Measure Fore Measure, Act II, Sc. I
118	Merchant of Venice, Act III, Sc. IV
119	Romeo and Juliet, Act IV, Sc. IV
120	Love's Labours Lost, Act V, Sc. II

Stationary Exercise Bicycles

One of the problems with cycling as a form of exercise in **"our brisk and giddy-paced times"** [121] is finding a safe, convenient location to ride. It is not uncommon for people to load their bike into their car and drive to a location where they feel safe riding.

"The heavens give safety to your purposes!"[122]

Even following this somewhat paradoxical behavior, and no matter how safety conscious we may be, there is still an element of risk posed by the presence of automobile traffic. In response to this concern, in recent years all manner of indoor exercise equipment, stationary exercise bikes, or ergometers, have become commonplace.

"shut the gates for safety of ourselves"[123]

Prices for stationary household bikes begin at about one hundred dollars with the highest quality trainers exceeding three hundred and fifty dollars. The stationary bike allows you to gain all of the cardiorespiratory benefits of cycling without having to worry about dealing with traffic, stray dogs, and other dangers.

"When least in company, prosper well in this" [124]

The popularity of indoor cycling is because you can exercise in privacy, any time, regardless of the weather, and you can read, watch TV, or listen to music at the same time! The problem with indoor cycling is that many people find riding a stationary bike, in one location, extremely boring and **"will stupefy and dull the sense!"** [125]

Regardless of which cycling approach you choose, the same principles of continuous training apply. The intensity should be sufficient to elevate the heart rate to between sixty percent and ninety percent of maximum, and the activity should be maintained for more than thirty minutes. This approach to bicycle training should improve cardiorespiratory endurance, contribute to muscle augmentation, skeletal system and joint flexibility, and body composition.

121	Twelfth Night, Act II, Sc. II
122	Measure for Measure, Act I Sc. I
123	King Henry VI, part III, Act IV, Sc. VII
124	Twelfth Night Act I Sc. IV
125	Cymbeline, Act I, Sc. V

"Needful Counsel To Our Business"[126]

Exercise Shoes and Fit Feet

"old shoes; when they are in great danger" [127]

The human foot has remained structurally unchanged for tens of thousands of years. **"Here's a strange alteration!"** [128] In contrast, sport and athletic *shoes* have changed and improved incredibly during the last thirty-five years and thereby have functionally and structurally exceeded the strength and integrity of the human foot. Fitness activity shoes too, have undergone exceptional improvements, and modifications. Shoe technology and construction have exceeded the human foot in its ability to withstand, produce, and handle forces associated with physical fitness endeavors. Therefore, people who engage in physical activity are more vulnerable to a wide range of both chronic and acute injuries " **... the feet were lame and could not bear."** [129] These difficulties are as likely to result from the superior shoes as well as from any unskilled movements or accidents.

"The service of the foot" [130]

The athletic and fitness shoe manufacturing industry has developed extremely sophisticated products expressly designed and produced for a wide variety of fitness activity options. In simpler times, if a person wanted shoes for physical activity or sports they simply had to decide on high-top or low-top, black or white.

Today we are **"full-replete with** [shoe] **choice**[s] **of all delights."** [131] Shoes for a wide variety of purposes and functions with all manner of features for fitness and sport have increased beyond belief. A whole new language has developed relative to activity and sport shoes. Words like toe box, outsole, external stabilizer, and Achilles pad are confusing to a person who simply wants to buy a pair of shoes because they are a pleasing color or attractive style and they just want shoes for play or exercise. Most people are simply interested in finding a reasonably priced shoe that will last, provide good support, and comfort. However, we frequently end up with a technically sophisticated shoe that is far better than our feet, our body and often our budgets. Sales people in quality athletic shoe stores are knowledgeable and definitely can help select the correct and appropriate shoe.

126	King Lear, Act II, Sc. I
127	Julius Caesar, Act I, Sc. I
128	Coriolanus, Act IV, Sc. V
129	As You Like It Act III, Sc. II
130	Coriolanus, Act III, Sc. I
131	King Henry VI, part I, Act V, Sc. V

"This advice is free I give and honest." [132]

All this considered, what is a person supposed to do when purchasing shoes for activity and fitness?

"give room! and foot it" [133]

There should be one half to three fourths of an inch between the tips of the toes and the front of the shoe. Shoe width should be suitable for the width of the foot. The shoe that accommodates these length and width considerations, regardless of color, style, or brand, is the one that should be purchased. There should be room for you to wiggle your toes in fitness and activity shoes. The best way to make sure shoes fit properly is to have both feet accurately measured and then try on both shoes that are being considered. It is advisable to try shoes on late in the day rather than early to allow for size fluctuations from normal swelling. We need to be certain that the shoes are suitable for both feet because it is not unusual to have feet that are not identical in size, shape, or dimension.

"it hath the worser sole. This shoe, with the hole" [134]

The soles of fitness activity shoes should first and foremost provide a protective cushioning against the impact force of the foot and ground. Additionally, the sole of activity fitness shoes should be **"constant in a wondrous excellence."** [135] That is, the soles should be tough, enduring, provide good traction, and resist wear. The soles of most fitness activity shoes are composed of a number of layers, with three being the usual minimum number. Of the three layers, one is usually intended to absorb the force of the foot strike under the heel. A second layer is intended to pad and protect the foot and toes and at least one other layer is usually made of a hard rubber and is this part of the sole that contacts the ground.

The ruthless flint doth cut my tender feet" [136]

Running shoes should be constructed specifically for the absorption and reduction of forces **"upon the foot of motion"** [137] that result from the heel strike against the ground. This is necessary because the repeated pounding of the foot and heel against the ground with each running stride may lead to overuse-type injuries which can adversely effect not only the foot but also the ankles and knees.

"One woe doth tread upon another's heel" [138]

Heel inserts are sometimes used to further protect and minimize impact forces on the heels,

---

132	Othello, Act II, Sc. III
133	Romeo and Juliet, Act I, Sc. V
134	The Two Gentlemen of Verona, Act II, Sc. III
135	Sonnet CV
136	King Henry VI, part II, Act II, Sc. IV
137	Macbeth, Act II, Sc. III
138	Hamlet, Act IV, Sc. VII

feet, ankles, and knees while running. Additionally, flared heel construction on running fitness shoes can stabilize the foot and minimize any tendency of the foot to roll from side to side during the foot strike. One additional consideration relating to the lower part of the shoe is arch support. An arch support should be soft and yet rugged and should, as is the case with all inner parts of a fitness shoe, seamlessly merge with the sole and upper parts of the shoe. The tops or upper parts of fitness activity shoes should be made of some combination of nylon, leather and rubber. The upper part of the shoe should be lightweight, capable of quick drying, and well ventilated. The upper part of the shoe should have some extra padding in the area of the Achilles tendon just above the heel.

"Being nimble-footed, he hath outrun us" [139]

When purchasing shoes for fitness activities, remember that the correct shoe, a suitable quality shoe, can facilitate activity and prevent injuries. Expensive shoes may be too sophisticated, structurally advanced, and contribute to aches, pains, and injury. Conversely, inexpensive shoes may be poorly constructed, structurally unsound, and likewise harm the feet, cause soreness and result in injury. Certain brand names, fashion and celebrity endorsements should never be factors when selecting shoes. Some fitness shoes may cost as little as thirty to forty dollars while others, because of style, name recognition, celebrity endorsements and quality may cost as much as one hundred seventy-five dollars. We must remember that fitness activity shoes can and should facilitate exercise and minimize pain, discomfort and the potential for injuries. Therefore, the shoe that is ultimately purchased should be appropriate for the activity and priced sensibly based on its function and quality.

"Sharp misery had worn him to the bones" [140]

There is always the danger that people who have purchased and used proper shoes will keep and use them too long. Shoes wear out! A worn shoe has many of the potential dangers that improper or incorrect shoes have. Do not let yourself become so attached to an activity shoe that you cannot get rid of it when it is old and worn out!

Exercise Clothing

"And do you now put on your best attire?" [141]

𝔍n its simplest sense, exercise clothing should be comfortable, functional and allow free and unrestrained motion. Interestingly, exercise and activity clothing has become **"the fashion of the world"** [142] a clothing statement that says **"youth and bloom of**

---

139   The Two Gentlemen of Verona, Act V, Sc. III
140   Romeo and Juli. Act V, Sc. I
141   Julius Caesar, Act I, Sc. I
142   Much Ado About Nothing, Act I, Sc. I

lustihood," [143] even if a person is not.

"His garments are rich, but he wears them not handsomely." [144]

There are some important considerations that should be understood before selecting fitness and activity clothing. Weather conditions should always be considered before selecting the clothing which will be worn when exercising. **"Fie! this is hot weather."** [145] When exercising in hot humid weather, exercise clothing should allow for maximum dissipation of body heat while minimizing the heat gained from the environment. By far, the most efficient means of heat loss involves the process of perspiration and its evaporation. If sweat does not or cannot evaporate, if your clothes become drenched with sweat, the body's ability to reduce body temperature or dissipate heat is greatly diminished.

"our garments, being, as they were, drenched" [146]

Therefore, exercise clothing must be lightweight, capable of drying quickly, and capable of letting moisture evaporate off the skin. There are other means the body possesses for eliminating heat but perspiring and evaporation are the most important. **"Take heed, lest by your heat you burn yourselves."** [147] Clothing that is worn during exercise should not interfere with these cooling processes. Cotton shirts such as tank tops allow for the greatest measure of evaporation.

"I'll sigh celestial breath, whose gentle wind Shall cool the heat of the descending sun." [148]

Radiation is another mechanism the body uses to diminish body heat. It can, under some environmental circumstances, increase body temperature. Heat from the sun or other hot surfaces like pavement may cause the body to gain heat. Clothing should be a light color to reflect as much heat as possible. It is also advisable to wear a hat to ward off radiant heat coming from the sun. Additionally, it is desirable that the hat be made of some type of mesh fabric to allow heat energy to evaporate from the head.

"my very lips might freeze to my teeth, my tongue to the roof of my mouth" [149]

When exercising in cold, wet, or windy weather special activity clothing should be worn in order to create and maintain an environment immediately around the body that is comfortable, and conducive of continued activity. Exercising in **"the to-and-fro-**

143	Much Ado About Nothing, Act V, Sc. I
144	The Winter's Tale, Act IV, Sc. IV
145	King Henry IV, part II, Act III, Sc. II
146	The Tempest, Act II, Sc. I
147	King Henry VI, part II, Act V, Sc. I
148	Venus and Adonis, Stanza 32
149	The Taming of the Shrew, Act IV, Sc. I

conflicting wind and rain" [150] is normally not a major threat to health. This, because muscle activity produces heat which can maintain body temperature. Because heat is produced as a by-product of muscle work, the clothing that is worn should be lightweight, comfortable, not overly insulating and allow easy and free body movement. Additionally, the clothing should be able to prevent chilling and be capable of maintaining the body temperature within acceptable ranges.

"A chilling sweat o'er-runs my trembling joints"[151]

Clothing material should allow for the passage of moisture and heat away from the body. It is not a good practice to wear cotton immediately next to the skin. This, because if cotton gets wet, either from the weather or perspiration, it loses its insulating value. If moisture is prevented from dissipating through the activity clothing then the moisture may accumulate on the skin or in the clothing and contribute to a chilling effect. **"twill endure wind and weather."** [152] Dampness, in combination with cold and wind, can contribute significantly to the possible development of hypothermia. Cold weather activity clothing should be made up of thin layers that can be easily added to or removed as temperatures change. The adjustment of clothing layers can reduce sweating and minimize the likelihood that clothing may become wet. Before beginning activity, during rest periods, and after exercise, a warm-up or sweat suit should be worn to prevent chilling.

"you angry stars of heaven! Wind, rain, and thunder, remember, earthly man Is but a substance that must yield to you" [153]

Therefore, while exercising in rainy or windy conditions a person might be unable to maintain acceptable body temperature or achieve acceptable heat production which may increase discomfort and force the person to cease activity.

"cold, indeed; and labour lost" [154]

Finally, in cold, wet and windy weather a hat or cap should be worn. This because in a cold environment as much as forty percent of the body's heat may be dissipated and lost through the head and neck.

150	King Lear Act III, Sc. I
151	Titus Andronicus, Act II, Sc. III
152	Twelfth Night, Act I, Sc. V
153	Pericles, Prince of Tyre, Act II, Sc. I
154	Merchant of Venice, Act II, Sc. VII

Final Thoughts

"My words fly up, my thoughts remain below: Words without thoughts never to heaven go" [155]

There are a hundred and sixty-eight hours in a week. Most of us spend forty to fifty of these hours each week *working*. Additionally, approximately fifty hours each week are spent sleeping. Of the remaining hours, if we are at all concerned with our health and fitness we must set aside thirty minutes per day—approximately three and a half hours per week—for physical activity. It must be understood that this amount of time is the absolute minimum! Ideally, greater time for physical activity would be far more beneficial.

"This thing's to do;' Sith I have cause and will and strength and means To do't" [156]

The activities and exercises we engage in should be comfortable and enjoyable. **"Pleasure and action make the hours seem short."** [157] Regular, constant, and deliberate physical activity and an active lifestyle will contribute significantly to physical fitness.

"Bend thoughts and wits to achieve"[158]

When we begin an exercise program we should possess clear goals that are realistic and achievable. The exercise that we select for ourselves should be viewed as pleasurable and enjoyable not a burden or chore. Physical activity should be a celebration of life, not torturous or painful. Next, remember that your weight on a scale or reflection in the mirror should not be the primary goal or principle indicator of exercise success.

"excitements of my reason and my blood" [159]

It is not uncommon when beginning a work-out to possess and experience great anticipation, and a high degree of motivation. Once the initial excitement wanes, it is not unusual for people to consciously or unconsciously begin making excuses, reduce activity effort, or even quit exercising altogether.

"And fix most firm thy resolution." [160]

155	Hamlet, Act III, Sc. III
156	Hamlet Act IV, Sc. IV
157	Othello, Act II, Sc. III
158	The Taming of the Shrew, Act I, Sc. I
159	Hamlet, Act IV, Sc. IV
160	Othello, Act V, Sc. I

Setting goals that are realistically achievable will help prevent this from occurring. Another phenomenon we must guard against is pushing ourselves too hard. By taking a gradual approach to physical activity, behavior and attitudes are more likely to become a habit. Outrageous overnight results promised by countless magazine articles, new product claims, and professed fitness authorities also contribute to the high exercise dropout rates. This because they build false expectations and often impose rigid standards that most people cannot meet. Emphasizing unrealistic health benefits and claims of fantastic body changes do not sustain motivation or help us stick with programs that do not produce the promised results.

Regular physical activity not only promotes fitness, but also boosts longevity. Most people possess a notion of the benefits of exercise, but turning these notions into *action* can be quite another matter. We frequently make excuses for not exercising but we must appreciate its value and commit to a lifestyle that is lively and physically active. **"Excuses shall not be admitted; there is no excuse."**[161] Getting started is probably the most difficult part of a fitness program. Select an activity, or activities that you enjoy and set aside time every day to exercise. It takes about two or three months for exercise and increased activity to become habitual and a regular part of a person's life. One additional consideration is that you are never too old to exercise, and it is never too late to begin. Commit yourself to improvement by starting your fitness program today.

"commit'st thy anointed body to the cure" [162]

---

161 King Henry IV, part II, Act V, Sc. I
162 King Richard II, Act II, Sc.I

My Life, My Joy, My Food

Chapter V

NUTRITION, DIET, AND PHYSICAL FITNESS

"My life, my joy, my food, my all the world!" [1]

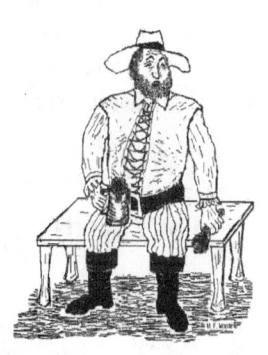

Diet and nutrition are probably as important to fitness as physical activity. The relationship, however, is an inverted one. People today should increase physical activity and consume a better diet which, **"in the fatness of these pursy[2] times,"** [3] means eat less. Stated even more simply, the way we live our lives in most industrialized societies gradually turns us into **"stuffed cloak-bag[s] of guts,"**[4] **"full of bread and sloth."** [5] We must learn to balance the ease and pleasures of contemporary eating with modern perceptions regarding the inconvenience and aggravations we commonly associate with exercise and physical activity. Most importantly, we must understand that there is no short-cut which leads to physical fitness. Certainly, there is no magic through the mouth and digestive system! Many people today are eager to believe that reduced food intake, unusual food combinations, secret enzymes, mega vitamin consumption, or special supplements will ultimately and quickly lead to fitness. This concept is ridiculous! **"To reason most absurd"** [6] and try to reduce our *thickened-up* bodies and diminish body weight, as is commonly the goal, reflects a significant misunderstanding of physical fitness, and ignores our body's requirement for essential nutrients.

---

1   King John, Act III, Sc. IV
2   bloated
3   Hamlet, Act III, Sc. IV
4   King Henry IV, part I Act II, Sc. IV
5   The Two Noble Kinsmen, Act I, Sc. I
6   Hamlet, Act I, Sc. II

> **"They are as sick that surfeit with too much as they that starve with nothing"** [7]

We all should eat wholesome foods which furnish us with appropriate nutrients so we may live, maintain good health, function and physiologically survive. Without proper nutrition, the body will not stay warm, build or repair tissue, maintain circulatory function, or efficiently perform the processes that are necessary for life. Poorly balanced or inadequate nutrition may ultimately result in deficiency diseases and various health problems. This is certainly the case in conditions like anorexia nervosa and bulimia. Health troubles may also result from the diets we choose for ourselves in an effort to achieve attractive shapes or pleasing physiques. Nutritional deficiencies resulting from various diet approaches for the purpose of achieving desirable body "shapes" often result in diminished vitamins and minerals, insufficient calories and incorrect and unhealthy nutrient quantities. When poor food choices are made, a person may feel satiated, may be making some progress toward their desired body shape but may simultaneously be getting inadequate calories, disproportionate or inadequate nutrients and be undernourished or even malnourished.

> **"O, I am slain! famine and no other hath slain me"** [8]

In Elizabethan times dining and nutritional considerations were very different than today. To begin with, the most important meal of the day was usually eaten at mid day. This was not too odd in itself, what was unusual was the sorts of things that were eaten. Included among foods commonly eaten, particularly by the more wealthy classes, were such items as pigeons, duck, crane, swan, stork and peacock.

> **"Some pigeons, Davy, a couple of short-legged hens, a joint of mutton, and any pretty little tiny kickshaws**[9] **... "** [10]

Additionally, fish of all sorts, as well as such sea creatures as porpoise, dolphin, otter, eel and seal were common fare. In fact, there were 153 designated "fish days" imposed by the church and government to discourage the eating of meats. Besides the preceding fare, oysters were plentiful and cheap and widely consumed. They were sold by street vendors and prepared in various ways. Finally, and traditionally, the meals of certainly the most prosperous citizenry but others too, ended with a course of sweets referred to as the "*banquet*".

The typical meal of these less prosperous citizens was much simpler, not as bizarre perhaps even boring, consisting mainly of breads, cheese, and only occasionally meats, usually mutton or fish. Vegetables were eaten reluctantly and primarily by those that could afford

---

7   The Merchant of Venice, Act I, Sc. II
8   King Henry VI, part II, Act IV, Sc. X
9   appetizer
10   King Henry IV, part II, Act V Sc. I

little else. Elizabethans were aware of potatoes but they were rarely consumed. Tomatoes, corn and various fruits which originated in the New World were often misunderstood, suspect and like potatoes very slow to be adopted in Elizabethan diets. By contrast blackberries, apples, figs, apricots and berries were common and widely consumed.

The beverage of choice for almost all meals, e.g. breakfast, lunch, and dinner was English ale. Wine was also commonly consumed, in large quantities, while coffee, tea, and chocolate beverages were still unknown.

In Shakespeare's time, malnutrition and deficiency diseases were fairly common, often the resulted of poverty, inefficient farming methods, inadequate food distribution, rustic lifestyles, feudal inefficient land usage, wars, and or famine.

Today it is widely understood that eating nutritious foods, in appropriate amounts, can help us avoid certain diseases, enhance body function and contribute to recovery from illness or physical injury. In present society, acquiring and eating adequate food is rarely, if ever, a problem. It is excess energy consumption that is the cause of most of our nutrition problems and that tend **"to overbulk us all."** [11] Conversely, eating foods which lack nutrition, or eating nutritious food in inappropriate quantities may increase the risk of disease, illness, and interfere with many cellular and bodily functions. *Malnutrition* still exists today.

"Consumed with that which it was nourish'd by"[12]

Thoughtless bad choices, buffet dining, "supersizing" and eating excesses generally are the cause of today's nutritional difficulties. Fast food, drive-through dining, snack foods, desserts, and empty calories conspire to make us malnourished, **"fat and greasy citizens."** [13] When thoughtless or uninformed food choices are made, a person may be getting adequate or even excessive calories yet still be malnourished.

"all viands that I eat do seem unsavoury" [14]

Complicating present day nutritional problems is the fact that the digestive system, appetite and nutrition preferences have evolved over millions of years of struggling to survive. In modern society nutritional choices are plentiful, extensive, and replete with **"inventions to delight the taste."**[15]

"More than a little is by much too much" [16]

---

11   Troilus and Cressida, Act I, Sc. III
12   Sonnet LXXIII
13   As You Like It, Act II, Sc. I
14   Pericles, Prince of Tyre, Act II, Sc. III
15   Pericles Prince of Tyre, Act I, Sc. IV
16   King Henry IV, part I, Act III, Sc. II

Good nutrition means providing the body, through correct eating and drinking, what it needs and in suitable amounts. The body needs carbohydrates, proteins, fats, vitamins, minerals, and water. All nutrients are required for good nutrition and must be present in correct amounts for proper body function. If our diet is deficient in any of the essential nutrients for an extended period of time, then our body's function, health and certainly physical fitness will deteriorate.

"I prithee go and get me some repast;
I care not what, so it be wholesome food" [17]

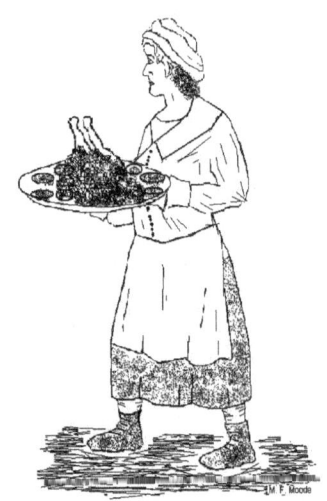

The nutritional problems that characterize most advanced societies today do not result from deficiencies but rather from excesses and overindulgence. Today's nutritional troubles are caused by overeating energy nutrients—carbohydrates, proteins, and fats eaten too often, too frequently and too easily for their pleasurable tastes or just because they are easily available. **"He hath put all my substance into that fat belly"**[18] When we eat appropriate amounts of carbohydrates, proteins, and fats, they are broken down and simplified through the digestive processes and essential nutrients are released into the body to supply the substances and energy the body needs. As we grow older, and as a result of sedentary lifestyles, our body's ability to use the energy present in dietary fat gradually diminishes. At the same time, our body's ability to store unused energy in the body's fat cells becomes more efficient. The effect of these natural phenomena can be reduced if we maintain a physically active lifestyle.

"unquiet meals make ill digestions" [19]

The energy released from the food we eat and used by the body is measured in kilocalories. A kilocalorie is the amount of energy needed to raise one kilogram of distilled water one degree Celsius. When discussing diet and energy nutrients, it has become quite common to use the term calorie instead of kilocalorie. Although this is technically not accurate, calorie is generally understood as the standard unit for measurement of the energy in nutrients. The body uses the energy released from carbohydrates, protein and fats to function and perform all cellular and life activities. An interesting aspect of today's energy preoccupation is that of all the energy we eat each day, approximately two thousand kilocalories, about seventy-five per cent of them or fifteen hundred kilocalories are expended just maintaining various life processes: heart beat, digestion, thinking, growing, breathing, etc. The remaining or unused

---

17   The Taming of the Shrew, Act IV, Sc. III
18   King Henry IV, part II, Act II, Sc. I
19   The Comedy of Errors, Act V, Sc. I

twenty-five per cent, approximately five hundred kilocalories, are available and may be expended effectively through muscular activity, or it may be saved and stored in our fat cells.

"I am weak with toil, yet strong in appetite" [20]

The expenditure of the remaining twenty-five per cent, approximately five hundred kilocalories is not as easy as most of us believe. With some slight variation, based on individual height and weight, consider that it would take about twenty minutes of continuous running or jumping rope to burn about one hundred and fifty kilocalories. Walking a brisk two miles or vigorous yard work similarly will consume about one hundred and fifty kilocalories. These types of activities are not that unusual in most exercise programs.

"they would melt me out of my fat drop by drop" [21]

The problem is that when this extra physical activity is completed, there still remains three hundred and fifty unused kilocalories that ultimately will end up being stored as body fat.

"Doth fat me with the very thoughts of it!" [22]

Digestion

"A good digestion to you all" [23]

Before considering the relationship between fitness and nutrition, perhaps we should take a moment to consider the process of extracting nutrients from the food we eat. Digestion is the physiological process by which food is broken down into its basic nutritional compounds and absorbed into the blood for transportation to the body's cells. Digestion begins in the mouth by the mechanical simplification of food by the teeth in the process of chewing. Additionally, the chemical activity of saliva also contributes to the break down and simplification of food in the mouth. Next, digestion continues as food remains in the **"fair round belly"** [24] where more powerful acids chemically break down the food even further.

> "That I receive the general food at first,
> Which you do live upon; and fit it is,
> Because I am the store-house and the shop
> Of the whole body: but, if you do remember,
> I send it through the rivers of your blood,
> Even to the court, the heart, to the seat o' the brain" [25]

20	Cymbeline, Act III, Sc. VI
21	Merry Wives of Windsor, Act IV, Sc. V
22	Titus Andronicus, Act III, Sc. I
23	King Henry VIII, Act I Sc. IV
24	As You Like It, Act II, Sc. VII
25	Coriolanus, Act I, Sc. I

Eventually, the mechanically simplified and chemically reduced nutrients exit the **"most grave belly"** [26] and begin to travel through the small intestine. Digestive enzymes and acids liquefy food, and nutrients are absorbed through the walls of the intestines into the circulatory system. All the while peristaltic muscle contractions push everything along the digestive tract. Once digested, and circulating in the blood, carbohydrates, proteins, and fats are capable of providing energy for the body's needs.

"blood to blush through lively veins" [27]

However, the energy derived from these nutrients is not equally great or equally usable by the body's cells. Additionally, cells of the body use various components associated with carbohydrates, proteins, and fats for building, repairing, regulating and assisting various cell functions and body needs. The unusable nutrients and parts of foods that are not absorbed continue to move down the intestinal tract and are finally eliminated from the body. This physiological process of digestion and absorption has served mankind effectively and well for as long as humans have existed.

"chew'd, swallow'd and digested"[28]

The incredible, resilient, human digestive system has enabled and contributed to humanity's survival and yet through all human history it has often been and continues to be abused, and neglected. Digestion is a remarkable physiological process. In our present **"unquiet wrangling days"** [29] digestion is, along with appetite, often demonized and blamed for society's increasing weight problems, deteriorating health, and negative self images. We are often preoccupied with digestive function and frequently blame digestion as the cause of our ever-increasing body fat and diminishing body composition.

"Now, good digestion wait on appetite" [30]

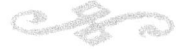

Knowledgeable Nutrition Choices

"let us dine and never fret" [31]

In Elizabethan England, food selection was much less complicated than today. People in Shakespeare's time ate what they gathered, grew, hunted or found. Foods were simple and simply prepared.

26	Coriolanus, Act I, Sc. I
27	Sonnet LXVII
28	King Henry V, Act II, Sc. II
29	King Richard III, Act II, Sc. IV
30	Macbeth, Act III Sc. IV
31	The Comedy of Errors, Act II, Sc. I

"twill fill your stomachs; please you eat of it" [32]

Obtaining food has been the primary occupation of humanity for virtually all time. Throughout most of that time there was little choice or selection in types of foods, preparation, snacks, treats, appetizers, entrees, or desserts. People ate what they had! It was basic, plain and usually contained at least rudimentary nutrition.

"wouldst thou have me go and beg my food?" [33]

The quest for food almost always involved a degree of physical effort and the body's energy inputs were closer to energy outputs than today. Hunting and gathering food today is *effortless*! This fact alone explains why it is so common today to corrupt the body's normal composition and accumulate excess body fat. Additionally, our energy-saving, automated, power-assisted lifestyles account for the difficulty we have trying to reduce or decrease body fat. Complicating our nutrition choices is the fact that food options are more varied than they have ever been. To deal with these emerging nutritional problems, in the late 1940's, early 1950's, the U.S. Department of Agriculture introduced a system and guide for grouping foods and ensuring a healthy variety. The original food guide was the *Basic Seven* food groups which ultimately by the mid 1950's evolved into the *Basic Four*. By the early 1990's a new type of food guide based on five major food groups emerged and was known as the *Food Guide Pyramid*. Since the introduction of the Food Guide Pyramid a number of variations of the original pyramid have been developed. There currently exists Food Guide Pyramids specifically for the elderly, young children, native Americans, Asians and even vegetarians.

"Thy pyramids built up with newer might" [34]

The Food Pyramid is based on key nutrients in foods, emphasizing general types of food items rather than specific nutrients. The base of the pyramid depicts the types and serving amounts of foods that should constitute the greatest portion of a person's diet. These items include grains, cereal, bread, rice, pasta. Foods that are in the mid-portion of the pyramid are items that should be included in moderate amounts such as meats, poultry, fish and dairy products. Additionally, valuable food items such as fruits and vegetables are also included in the middle of the food pyramid. Finally, at the top of the pyramid are foods that should be consumed only sparingly and include such foodstuffs as fats, oils, sweets. The more recently developed Food Guide Pyramids besides recognizing age, cultural and other societal differences include recommendations for daily physical activity. The value of the food pyramid as a guide to good nutrition must be questioned. This, because as a population we seem to be turning into pyramids rather than eating better or exercising more. **"Palaces and pyramids do slope"** [35] as unfortunately do most of our bodies

---

32	Titus Andronicus, Act V, Sc. III
33	As You Like It, Act II, Sc. III
34	Sonnet CXXIII
35	MacBeth, Act IV, Sc. I

in a downward direction toward our prominent abdomens, broad hips, and fat thighs **"all filled up with guts and midriff."** [36]

Another source of nutritional information is the *Nutrition Facts Panel* required on most food packages. These labels are required on foods that contain more than one ingredient, and are usually processed types of foods. The Nutrition Facts Panel displays the amount of fat, percent saturated fat, cholesterol, sodium, fiber, vitamins A and C, calcium, iron and calories present in packaged foods. Food manufacturers may provide additional information about other nutrients if they choose. However, if a nutritional claim is made on a product's package, the appropriate nutrient content must be listed.

Non-Energy Nutrients

Water

"Here's that which is too weak to be a sinner, honest water, which ne'er left man in the mire" [37]

The human body is approximately sixty-five percent water. We should drink at least six to eight glasses of water each day to replenish the water the body needs whether we are physically active or sedentary.

"By Providence divine. Some food we had and some fresh water"[38]

Of all the essential nutrients, water is the most important. We can function for only a short time, a couple of days at most, without water. Conversely, we may continue to live and function for extended periods of time without other nutrients. It may take weeks or even months to adversely effect life functions, develop deficiency diseases, or even die from a lack of other nutrients. Water is an essential component of blood and facilitates functioning of the circulatory and lymphatic systems. It enhances the transport of oxygen and nutrients to all the cells in the body and removal of wastes from cells. All body fluids depend on water, and water contributes to the growth, function and existence of all cells, all tissues, and all the organs of the body.

" ... the water itself was a good healthy water"[39]

---

36   Henry IV, part I, Act III, Sc. III
37   Timon of Athens, Act I, Sc. II
38   The Tempest, Act I, Sc. II
39   King Henry IV, part II, Act I, Sc. II

While water has no caloric value and therefore is not an energy nutrient, with insufficient water the energy which is part of other nutrients will not be digested, absorbed, utilized or eliminated properly or effectively. The body's water demands are increased if a person is engaged in frequent and vigorous physical activity or exercise. Therefore, water should be consumed constantly during exercise or physical activity.

"When they are thirsty, fools would fain have drink." [40]

When a person engaged in activity is conscious of thirst, in terms of continued performance it is too late! When feelings of thirst have risen to a conscious level, strength and performance will have deteriorated perhaps as much as ten percent.

"With satiety seeks to quench his thirst." [41]

Water is essential to continued and high level performance. Fluids are replenished in the body by drinking liquids, preferably those liquids which contain no caffeine or alcohol. Caffeine and alcohol both possess a diuretic effect and increase the output of urine and thus dehydrate the body. Besides drinking fluids to supply sufficient water, many foods are also a good source of water. Vegetables and fruits, depending on how they are prepared, may be eighty to ninety-five percent water. Meats, poultry, and fish may be as much as fifty percent water. Carbohydrates such as grains, rice and oats contain approximately thirty-five percent water.

Fiber

"to dine and sup with water and bran" [42]

Fiber, which is an indigestible substance, is found only in plants and provides no energy or physiological structural components and yet is essential to good nutrition, and ultimately to good health. There are two types of dietary fiber which are classified as either soluble or insoluble.

"Of wheat, rye, barley, vetches, oats and pease" [43]

Soluble fiber is in such foods as oats, barley, beans, peas, apples, strawberries, and citrus fruits. It functions to mix with food in the stomach and minimize the absorption of undesirable substances. Soluble fiber binds with dietary cholesterol and facilitates its elimination from the body. This function of fiber in the digestion system reduces the

---

40 Love's Labour's Lost, Act V, Sc. II
41 The Taming of the Shrew, Act I, Sc. I
42 Measure Fore Measure Act IV, Sc. III
43 The Tempest, Act IV, Sc. I

cholesterol rich **"unreprievable condemned blood"** [44] from circulating in the bloodstream where it accumulates on the inner walls of arteries, contributes to high blood pressure, and increases the risk of heart disease, and strokes.

Insoluble fiber, which is found in vegetables, whole-grain products, and bran, provides roughage that assists the digestion system in the elimination of unusable nutrients. Generally, the body does not consume or absorb insoluble fiber. It serves the body by mechanically enhancing and facilitating digestion function thereby reducing the risk of colon cancer, as well as other cancers.

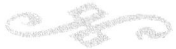

Vitamins and Minerals

" ... in league, coupled and linked together" [45]

Both vitamins and minerals are needed by the body in small amounts to facilitate the thousands of chemical reactions necessary to maintain life and good health. Neither vitamins nor minerals possess or furnish energy in any amount. Many of the actions that are facilitated by vitamins and minerals are linked with one action triggering another. If some vitamins or minerals are missing or deficient then one or more essential connections along the metabolic chain may not occur. This could lead to potentially devastating health effects.

"As if those organs had deceptious functions" [46]

Vitamins and minerals have many significant differences. Among their many functions, vitamins enhance the body's use of carbohydrates, proteins, and fats. Further, they are **"the essential vesture[s] of creation"** [47] in the formation of blood cells, hormones, nervous system neurotransmitters, and the genetic material deoxyribonucleic acid (DNA).

Vitamins are classified as either fat soluble or water soluble. Fat-soluble vitamins, which include vitamins A, D, E, and K, are usually absorbed with the help of foods that contain fat. Fat containing these vitamins is broken down by bile, a liquid released by the liver, and the body then absorbs the simplified substances and vitamins. Excess amounts of fat-soluble vitamins are stored in the body's fat, liver, and kidneys. **"More than a little is by much too much."** [48] Because these vitamins are stored in the body, they do not need to be consumed every day to meet the body's needs. "Why then, can one desire too

---

44	King John, Act V, Sc. VII
45	King John, Act III, Sc. I
46	Troilus and Cressida, Act V, Sc. II
47	Othello Act II, Sc. I
48	King Henry IV, part I, Act III, Sc. II

much of a good thing?" [49] Excessive amounts of fat soluble vitamins can become a serious health problem and may be life threatening.

Water-soluble vitamins, which include vitamins C (ascorbic acid), B1 (thiamine), B2 (riboflavin), B3 (niacin), B6, B12, and folic acid, cannot be stored and rapidly leave the body in urine if taken in greater quantities than the body needs. Foods that contain water-soluble vitamins need to be eaten every day in order to meet the body's demands.

"Is more than my o'er-press'd defense can bide" [50]

In addition to other functions, the vitamins A (beta-carotene), C, and E function as antioxidants. Antioxidants, it is believed, play a unique and vital role in resisting the potential harmful chemicals which result from metabolism that are known as free radicals.

"Which harm within itself so heinous is" [51]

If free radicals are allowed to remain unchecked in the body it is believed that they injure cells, impair cell membranes, damage DNA and increase vulnerability to various cancers. Free radicals may also facilitate the changes of harmless environmental substances that are common in the body, into cancer-facilitating substances.

Minerals are tiny inorganic elements **"whose want gives growth to. . . . imperfections"** [52] because they are vitally important for healthy growth of teeth and bones. They also help in such cellular activities as enzyme action, muscle contraction, nervous system functioning, and blood clotting. Mineral nutrients are classified as major elements (calcium, chlorine, magnesium, phosphorus, potassium, sodium, and sulfur) and trace elements (chromium, copper, fluoride, iodine, iron, selenium, and zinc).

Vitamins and minerals not only help the body perform its various life functions, but also contribute to the defenses against a wide range of diseases and health problems. For example, vitamin C is important in maintaining our bones and teeth; scurvy, a disorder that attacks the gums, skin, and muscles, occurs in its absence. Diets lacking vitamin B1, which supports neuromuscular function, can result in beriberi, a disease characterized by mental confusion, muscle weakness, and inflammation of the heart. Adequate intake of folic acid by pregnant women is critical to avoid nervous system defects in the fetus. The mineral calcium plays a critical role in building and maintaining strong bones; without it, children develop weak bones and adults experience the progressive loss of bone mass known as osteoporosis, which increases their risk of bone fractures.

49	As You Like It, Act IV, Sc. I
50	Sonnet CXXXIX
51	King John, Act III, Sc. I
52	King Henry V, Act V, Sc. II

Energy Nutrients

Carbohydrates

"Feed'st thy light'st flame with self-substantial fuel"[53]

Carbohydrates furnish four calories of energy per gram and are the body's preferred source of energy. We should consume fifty-five percent of our total food intake in the form of carbohydrate. There are two types of carbohydrates: simple and complex. Complex carbohydrates may be either digestible, starches, or non-digestible, fiber. Complex carbohydrates are found in whole-grain breads, cereals, pasta, corn, beans, peas, vegetables, rice and potatoes. Besides being excellent sources of energy, complex carbohydrates are often good sources of vitamins, some minerals, as well as water. Foods that contain starch and naturally occurring sugars are complex, and their molecular structure requires that the body break them down into their simplest sugar form as glucose. The body digests and absorbs complex carbohydrates at a slow rate which helps maintain a reasonable level of glucose in the blood over a long period of time.

"Sweet, sweet, sweet poison for the age's tooth"[54]

In Shakespeare's time, people of all classes loved their foods sweet. In fact, sugar was considered somewhat of an aphrodisiac. It was common to cook all sorts of food with sugary coatings. Even wine was frequently augmented with a generous ration of sugar. So popular were sugars in Elizabethan times that people's teeth were characterized by disease, decay, and dark stains.

"Is wasteful and ridiculous excess." [55]

Simple carbohydrates are naturally occurring sugars and are present in fruits, vegetables, milk products, honey, maple sugar, and sugar cane. **"If ... sugar be a fault, God help the wicked!"** [56] Simple carbohydrates are refined sugars that are extremely pleasing to the taste and are frequently added to foods. It is not uncommon for many processed foods to be "*enriched*" with simple carbohydrates. Simple carbohydrates should make up no more that ten percent of a person's diet. This, because simple carbohydrates contain little significant nutritional value. Simple carbohydrates are easily digested and are quickly absorbed by the body. Many processed foods not only contain high levels of simple carbohydrates, they also tend to be high in fat and salt. Though sometimes enriched with vitamins, processed

---

53   Sonnet I
54   King John, Act I, Sc. I
55   King John, Act IV, Sc. II
56   King Henry IV, part I, Act II, Sc. IV

foods are generally high in calories, sugars, fats, and lack essential nutrients. These are frequently referred to as *"junk foods"* or *"empty calories."*

". . . .the last taste of sweets, is sweetest last" [57]

Through the digestive process, carbohydrates are broken down into glucose molecules which are absorbed into the bloodstream through the walls of the intestines. When glucose is absorbed through the walls of the intestines it is converted to blood sugar or glycogen. Glucose is the preferred source of energy used by all body cells. Glycogen is the body's storage, transport and auxiliary energy source. It is accessed and converted back into glucose when it is needed for more energy. An adequate amount of glucose protects and preserves protein for other more critical functions, and carbohydrates are the only fuel for operation of the central nervous system.

In the blood, some glycogen goes immediately to work providing energy for the nervous system, while the rest is transported to the liver or muscles for storage. Any excess glycogen is converted and stored as fat within body's fat cells. Among today's **"fat and greasy citizens"** [58] this is often the fate of the excessive carbohydrates which are eaten and not consumed or expended by the body's muscles or other systems.

"Is wasteful and ridiculous excess." [59]

Fiber, the other common type of complex carbohydrate is composed of a number of indigestible substances such as gums, pectins and muscilage. Fiber facilitates the efficient functioning of the digestive system and diminishes the risk of many health problems including certain cancers, cardiovascular disease, as well as various digestive disorders.

"a surfeit of the sweetest things
The deepest loathing to the stomach brings" [60]

Proteins

"Your greatest want is, you want much of meat" [61]

Proteins are complex nutrients made of smaller substances called amino acids. If consumed and used as a source of energy, proteins furnish energy in the amount of four

---

57 King Richard II, Act II, Sc. I
58 As You Like It, Act II, Sc. I
59 King Lear, Act Iv, Sc. II
60 A Midsummer Night's Dream, Act II, Sc. II
61 Timon of Athens Act, IV, Sc. III

calories per gram. These amino acids are nutritional compounds that the body prefers to use for building body tissues, repairing damaged cellular matter, and regulating body functions. The human body requires all twenty amino acids for sound nutrition and uses them as a source of energy only under unusual and undesirable circumstances. When we eat foods high in protein, the digestive tract simplifies the dietary protein into amino acids.

"this quintessence of dust" [62]

Everything from internal organs to hair, skin, hormones, enzymes, fingernails and muscles are made up of different combinations of amino acids. Amino acids expedite the body's various chemical reactions, promote function of the immune system, and facilitate oxygen transport in the blood. Protein does possess chemical energy, but the body uses protein for energy only if carbohydrates and fats are insufficient or not available. When used as a source of energy, protein greatly upsets the chemistry of the body. Additionally, using protein for energy limits the amounts that remain available for its primary and essential functions.

Of the twenty amino acids the body requires, eleven are produced within the body itself. The nine additional amino acids that are not produced by the body must be acquired by eating foods of animal origin in which they are contained. The nine amino acids, of animal origin, are collectively referred to as *essential* amino acids.

"I am a great eater of beef and I believe that does harm to my wit." [63]

Animal proteins, found in meat, eggs, milk, fish, and poultry, are considered complete proteins because they contain all of the essential amino acids. Some amino acids are present in plants. The amino acids which are found in vegetables, soy products, rice, grains, nuts, peas, and beans usually lack one or more of the essential amino acids. Plant proteins can be and often are combined in a person's diet to provide most, if not all, of the essential amino acids. It is generally recommended that protein intake make up approximately fifteen percent of a sound nutritional diet.

Fats

"As fat as butter" [64]

𝓕ats are the most concentrated of the energy nutrients and provide nine calories per gram. However, our bodies need only very small amounts of dietary fat and not all fats are equally desirable or beneficial. Generally, dietary fats are a problematic source of

---

62   Hamlet, Act II, Sc. II
63   Twelfth Night, Act I, Sc. III
64   King Henry IV, part I, Act II, Sc. IV

energy for the body. Dietary fat, as well as depot or stored body fat, may serve as sources of energy. When this happens it is an extremely complex physiological process and in **"this harsh world"** [65] rarely takes place. Fats do play an important role in cell fabrication, the structure of cell membranes, as well as in various tissue and blood functions. Dietary fat also facilitates the body's absorption vitamins A, D, E, and K. Stored or depot body fat is an evolutionary emergency source of energy. It cushions the body and vital organs, gives the body shape and form, and insulates us from extremes of heat and cold.

Fat is composed of fatty acids which are attached to a substance called glycerol. Dietary fats are classified as saturated, monounsaturated, and polyunsaturated depending on the structure of their fatty acids. Animal fats from eggs, dairy products, and meats are high in saturated fats and cholesterol. Vegetable fats which are present in avocados, olives, nuts, seeds, and certain vegetable oils are rich in monounsaturated and polyunsaturated fat.

"Your country's fat shall pay your pains the hire" [66]

Cholesterol is a special form of fat that serves a number of indispensable functions in the human body. The problem with excessive saturated fat in our diet is its relationship to cholesterol. A high level of cholesterol in the blood is a major factor in the development of cardiovascular disease. There is a contradiction though with cholesterol. Despite its bad reputation, the body needs cholesterol. It is essential in the creation of cell membranes and the formation of the protective sheaths that surround nerve fibers. It is important in the formation of many of the body's hormones and it contributes to the body's synthesis of vitamin D. Cholesterol is so important to our survival that the liver produces all of the cholesterol the body needs. Because of this, we do not need as much cholesterol in our diet as we typically consume. We manufacture all that we need, and then we supplement the internally-produced cholesterol with additional quantities of cholesterol that we consume in our contemporary diets.

Cholesterol is not soluble in water, therefore in order for cholesterol to travel through the blood, it must be transported through the body by special carriers, called lipoproteins. High-density lipoproteins (HDLs) remove cholesterol from the arteries, and return it to the liver. The liver excretes excess cholesterol as bile, a liquid acid essential to fat digestion. For this reason, HDL is called "good" cholesterol.

"give me swift transportance" [67]

Low-density lipoproteins (LDLs) and very-low-density lipoproteins (VLDLs) are transporters of the cholesterol that is loosely referred to as *bad*. Both LDLs and VLDLs transport cholesterol from the liver for delivery to body cells where it is needed. If there is too much cholesterol in the body, usually resulting from a bad diet, the LDLs and VLDLs

---

65 Hamlet, Act V, Sc. II
66 King Richard, Act V, Sc. III
67 Troilus and Cressida, Act III, Sc. II

dump cholesterol into the arteries forming plaque in the walls of the arteries, clogging them and setting the stage for cardiovascular disease. When eating foods of animal origin, which are the source of cholesterol and saturated fatty acids, we increase the level of both the (HDL) and (LDL) cholesterol carrying substances in our blood.

"I fear it is too choleric a meat" [68]

Saturated fatty acids are present in beef, butter, ice cream, cheese and virtually everything cooked in oil. Saturated fats increase the levels of cholesterol in the blood. These types of food should be a minor part of our diets-certainly no more than ten percent of a person's total caloric intake each day.

Monounsaturated fats which are in olive, canola, and peanut oils are good choices and help reduce the level of LDLs and VLDLs. These types of oils have the most positive effect on blood cholesterol. Polyunsaturated fat is present in margarine, sunflower, soybean, corn, and safflower oils. Polyunsaturated fat is a more positive and beneficial form of fat than saturated fat. However, as is the case with any nutrient, if it is consumed in excess it can have a negative effect on the body and over time adversely effect health.

Most Americans obtain fifteen to fifty percent of their daily calories from dietary fat. Diets with more than thirty percent of the calories from fat are dangerous. They put us at risk of heart disease, contribute to obesity, and diabetes. A diet high in both saturated and unsaturated fats has also been associated with greater risk of developing various cancers. Choosing a diet that is low in fat and cholesterol is critical to maintaining health and reducing the risk of life-threatening disease.

Eating Well—Nutritional Counsel

"Yourself shall give us counsel, feed, and sleep" [69]

People's tastes, eating habits, and foods vary greatly. Appetites and tastes are learned and have evolved differently among diverse cultures and different peoples. However modern research has determined that healthful eating is achieved by giving the body the nutrients it needs. These needs, with only slight variation are virtually identical for all people in all cultures throughout human history. The body's nutritional demands may be achieved by different foods but the precise nature and quantities of nutrients are universal. **"Your diet shall be in all places alike."** [70] In spite of this knowledge, eating and nutrition-related problems still exist and in some instances are very common and usually

---

68   The Taming of the Shrew, Act IV, Sc. III
69   Antony and Cleopatra, Act V Sc. II
70   Timon of Athens, Act III, Sc. VI

result from nutritional excesses. Chronic problems associated with extreme weight such as cardiovascular disease, diabetes, and various cancers are widespread in current society. The basic rules for healthy nutritious eating have been known and remained relatively unchanged for centuries. Among these rules and sound advice are the following:

"O, he hath kept an evil diet long" [71]

Good nutrition in modern times means perhaps first and foremost that we reduce our total fat intake to thirty percent or less of our total caloric intake. Dietary cholesterol, a form of fat, should be particularly monitored and limited. Organ cuts of meat like liver, kidney, intestines or brains, some shellfish, and egg yolks are all high in cholesterol and should be a very small portion of our diet. We should likewise limit our consumption of saturated fats which are found in dark-meat poultry, whole milk, dairy products and fatty meats, to less than one-third of total fat intake. Additionally, trans fat, a form of fat created when vegetable oils undergo the chemical process of hydrogenation, a procedure that extends its shelf life and is common in fast foods, convenience foods, packaged foods, and snacks, should be avoided. Both of these types of fats are closely associated with cholesterol and contribute to heart disease. In today's health-conscious diets it is very common for people to be aware of and eat more of the beneficial fats such as unsaturated and monounsaturated fat and avoid the unhealthy polyunsaturated fats. A diet that emphasizes lean cuts of meat, fish, skinless poultry, and low-fat or nonfat dairy products, reduces the total caloric intake without sacrificing important vitamins, minerals and fatty acids that are essential. Monounsaturated fats such as olive oil, peanut oil, and canola oil should be used to replace other fats in various spreads, dressings and if we must, for frying.

"Give it a plum, a cherry, and a fig" [72]

Eat plenty of fruits and vegetables every day. Additionally, increase your intake of rice, pasta, potatoes, bread and cereals and other complex carbohydrates. These complex carbohydrates are all good substitutes for fatty foods and excellent sources of various vitamins and minerals as well as dietary fiber. **"Four pound of prunes, and as many of raisins o' the sun."** [73] The importance of starches has long been known and they are now recognized as important as fiber in a healthy diet. Finally, pay particular attention to increasing green, yellow vegetables and citrus fruits.

---

71   King Rchard III, Act I, Sc. I
72   King John, Act II, Sc. I
73   The Winter's Tale Act IV, Sc. III

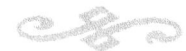

"meat sweet-savor'd in thy taste" [74]

Eat proteins only in moderate quantities. Proteins are the building blocks of the entire body and essential to the integrity of all cells. It is not uncommon today for people to eat more protein than the body actually needs. Because excessive protein, that is, amino acids, cannot be stored in the body, the body destroys these excess amino acids and excretes their by-products. Proteins should be about fifteen percent of the total food intake daily. However, the average amount of protein eaten today is considerably higher than these recommendations. It is widely known that there are no benefits and some problems associated with eating excessive amounts of protein. Too much protein consumption usually displaces and reduces the intake of other nutrients. Further, protein is usually associated with fat and therefore fat ingestion increases above recommended levels. The key advice here is eat lean meat, which is low in saturated fat and eat smaller portions. A simple guide to determine the desirable amount of meat to serve or eat is to not eat meat in quantities larger than a deck of cards or the palm of your hand.

"For thou exist'st on many a thousand grains" [75]

Fiber helps to keep our digestive systems working efficiently and regularly as well as providing us with a few nutrients. Fiber is a stringy, indigestible form of carbohydrate that is in fruits, vegetables, and grains. It keeps our digestive tract functioning efficiently. Additionally, it helps us lower cholesterol, avoid gallstones, minimize the chance of intestinal cancer, and facilitates our weight control efforts. Whole grain breads are full of fiber, as are brown rice, barley, lentils, beans and vegetables. You can further increase your fiber intake by choosing high fiber breakfast cereal, eating plenty of fruit and vegetables, whole grain rice, pasta, potatoes, and oats. If greatly increasing the amount of fiber in the diet, it is also important to enhance the amount of fluids consumed at the same time. **"Honest water, which ne'er left man i' the mire."** [76] Increasing fluid intake is desirable because excessive fiber may draw needed fluids from the digestive system and facilitate its elimination from the body. **"That's a fault that water will mend."** [77]

74	The Comedy of Errors, Act II, Sc. II
75	Measure Fore Measure, Act III, Sc. I
76	Timon of Athens, Act I, Sc. II
77	The Comedy of Errors, Act III, Sc. II

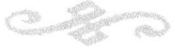

"Each hath his place and function" [78]

Vegetables, fruit and grains contain an abundance of vitamins and minerals. Vitamins play a part in virtually all body processes and functions. Vitamins are not manufactured in the body and therefore must be obtained through a nutritious diet. Contrary to common misconceptions, vitamins are not miraculous substances and perform no amazing or magical functions within the body. Additionally, there is no energy derived from vitamins. They simply serve to facilitate the many minute processes in the body that sustain life.

"To me and to my aid the blest infusions That dwell in vegetives, in metals. . . . " [79]

Minerals are tiny inorganic elements that are vitally important for healthy growth of teeth and bones. They also help in such cellular activity as enzyme action, muscle contraction, nervous system activity, and blood clotting. Calcium is the most common mineral in the body and deserves special attention in today's diet. Calcium is essential for maintaining adequate health of the bones, muscles, and teeth. Rich sources of calcium are low-fat or nonfat dairy products like skim milk, reduced-fat cheeses and dark-green vegetables such as broccoli and brussel sprouts. Calcium supplements are also popular, especially for individuals who cannot tolerate milk, sugar, or lactose.

"I drink, I eat, array myself, and live" [80]

No one food or food group can supply all of the essential nutrients that the body demands. Eating a wide variety of foods, prepared in different ways, will enhance the possibility that we will get a balanced nutritious diet. When preparing meats it is desirable and healthier to broil, barbecue grill, braise, or bake so that fat drips away and is diminished during the cooking process.

"What if this mixture do not work at all?" [81]

We must be aware that different forms of a food like pasta, bread or breakfast cereal, may all look and taste different but are all derived from the one basic grain, wheat. Because of this, the nutrients that these different foods supply will all be essentially the same. Different types of meat, fish and poultry, grains, and fruits and vegetables guarantee diversity in the diet and increase the chance that the body will receive all the nutrients it needs.

---

78   King Henry VI, part I, Act I, Sc. I
79   Pericles, Prince of Tyre, Act III, Sc. II
80   Measure Fore Measure, Act III, Sc. II
81   Romeo and Juliet, Act IV, Sc. III

"Honey, and milk, and sugar; there is three" [82]

Sugar is not essential for health or sound nutrition. We are born with a fondness and appetite for the taste of **"saucy sweetness."**[83] Sugar provides us with pleasing taste, empty calories and no nutrients. Our desire for sweet tastes was probably an evolutionary bit of good luck that helped humanity survive. This, because sweet tastes and smells usually indicated that something was safe for consumption. By contrast, foul smelling and bitter-tasting foods were usually toxic. The sweet taste of sugars in modest amounts adds to the flavor of foods and is a useful source of quick energy. **"I give thee this pennyworth of sugar."**[84] The problem, however, is that sugar in large quantities supplies great amounts of energy, and going unused as is often the case, it results in increased body fat. Additionally, simple sugars tend to deplete the body's vitamin stores, especially B complex vitamins. It can cause major fluctuations in blood glucose levels and lead to feelings of fatigue, headaches and as everyone knows sugars contribute to tooth decay.

"Why, this would make a man a man of salt"[85]

Our diets today are loaded with salt. A healthy diet should include no more than a total daily intake of about three grams or less of salt per day. Three grams is about the equivalent of a tea spoon. This amount of salt is naturally present in the foods we consume each day. Thus supplementing our foods by adding salt is undesirable. Diets high in salt are associated with high blood pressure. Hypertension or high blood pressure has been associated with salt intakes above six grams per day. **"The salt in them is hot."**[86] Salt in our diets adversely affects our ability to taste and enjoy foods generally. It is not until we reduce our intake of salt over a period of time that we are able to once again taste the true flavor of foods we eat.

"And salt too little which may season give"[87]

We should all limit the use of salt when cooking, and we should avoid adding salt to food at the table. Many foods, particularly commercially prepared foods, are heavily salted and should be consumed sparingly. As much as seventy-five per cent of our total salt intake may result from eating commercial foods. These foods include snack foods, deli meats,

---

82	Love's Labour's Lost, Act V, Sc. II
83	Measure Fore Measure, Act II, Sc. IV
84	King Henry IV, part I, Act II, Sc. IV
85	King Lear, Act IV, Sc. VI
86	King John, Act V, Sc. VII
87	Much Ado About Nothing, Act IV, Sc. I

most canned foods, many breads, condiments, and cereals. For good health and sound nutrition it is important that we reduce our salt intake. We should buy salt-reduced or no-added-salt products and cook without adding salt.

"feed upon such nice and waterish diet" [88]

Approximately sixty-five percent of the human body is water. Water is present in most foods, especially fruits and vegetables. The water in foods, combined with approximately six to eight glasses of water we should drink daily, ensures that we will get the two liters of fluid we need each day in order to keep the body hydrated and the kidneys working effectively. In hot weather, even more fluid is required. Alcohol and strong coffee do not count, as these act as diuretics and force the kidneys to excrete more fluid than normal.

"Thou art so fat-witted, with drinking of old sack" [89]

Alcohol is not a food, a nutrient, nor is it essential for health or good living. We should avoid drinking excess amounts of alcoholic beverages. There are recommended limits for alcohol intake and they are slightly different for men and women.

"expert in his drinking" [90]

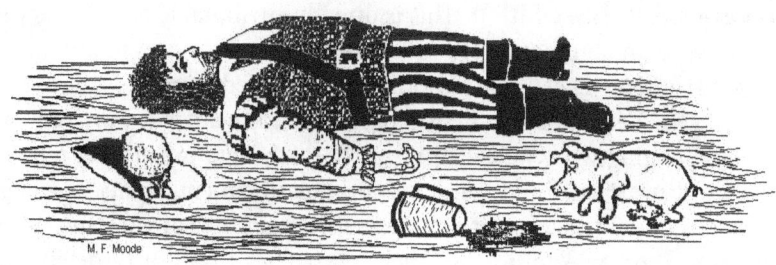

As a general rule and in the interest of good health, we should limit our drinking to no more than two cans of beer, two small glasses of wine, or two average-size cocktails at any given time. Additionally, it is most sound if these very moderate amounts of alcohol are consumed with meals **"let us therefore eat and drink."** [91] If alcohol is consumed, it

88   Othello, Act III, Sc. III
89   King Henry IV, part I Act I, Sc. II
90   Othello, Act II, Sc. III
91   Twelfth Night, Act II, Sc. III

should be consumed in small quantities and those quantities should be spread out over a period of hours. **"Distribution should undo excess."** [92] To drink large quantities of alcohol in a very short period of time is dangerous and unhealthy.

Like sugar, alcoholic beverages contain a lot of calories and no other nutrients. It also interferes with the body's ability to break down and use fat. Excessive drinking in the short term impairs judgment and over time it increases the risk for many diseases, including heart disease, liver disease, neurological disease, some forms of cancer, as well as many nutritional deficiencies.

Dieting, Physical Activity, and Weight Reduction

**"You'd be so lean, that blasts of January
Would blow you through and through."** [93]

In Shakespeare's time, body image, body fat, and body composition were minor considerations if contemplated at all. In contrast, **" ... we, which now behold these present days"** [94] often see in ourselves and in others a preoccupation and concern with negative body image and pessimistic views of body composition.

**"our virtues would be proud, if our
faults whipped them not"**[95]

It is common today to experience ever-increasing body fat throughout our lives. **"Doth fat me with the very thoughts of it!"**[96] This is directly attributable to sedentary lifestyles and effortless access to an abundance of foods. The usual solution to increasing body fat is generally to begin a diet. "Diet" has traditionally meant reducing the amounts of foods we put in our mouths. Very recently dieting has come to mean not only reducing food consumption but changing what we eat in terms of the body's nutritional requirements. Some diets involve eating unusual and unnatural combinations of nutrients. Diet approaches that advocate no carbohydrates, high protein, extreme quantities of vitamins, or no fat are increasingly common today. Additionally, diet approaches that utilize newly developed artificial substances that can block nutrient absorption or utilization and thereby hinder or minimize the body's ability to use or store excess nutritional energy are increasingly prevalent. It is not at all unusual today to be the prisoner of our own body weight concerns and body weight loss. We constantly seek to **"smite flat the thick rotundity o' the**

---

92   King Lear, Act IV, Sc. I
93   The Winter's Tale, Act IV, Sc. IV
94   Sonnet CVI
95   All's Well That Ends Well, Act IV, Sc. III
96   Titus Andronicus, Act III, Sc. I

world!" [97] Along with this preoccupation, if we could reduce weight and get skinny with no physical activity or exercise, we would do so without hesitation. There are those today who will be fulfilled and satisfied only if—

"famine is in thy cheeks, Need and oppression starveth in thine eyes" [98]

For good or ill we are blessed today with such fat reduction approaches as liposuction, body wraps, and diet pills. These actions and procedures are performed hundreds, perhaps thousands of times a day for cosmetic and egotistical reasons. **"O vanity of sickness! fierce extremes!"**[99] We all want to look and feel good—as long as it doesn't interfere with our eating pleasures and sedentary lifestyles!

"as heavy as my weight should be" [100]

Studies on managing body composition point to the overwhelming success of combining reasonable eating with regular physical activity rather than relying on the latest *miraculous, revolutionary, exotic foreign,* diet procedures!

The importance of regular physical activity in managing body fat and lean tissues is universally acknowledged. While reducing the amount of food we eat may help us lose weight, physical activity is necessary to maintain body composition throughout our lives. Physically active lifestyles and exercise are the keys to preserving muscle, maintaining a high metabolic rate, and thus, burning excess calories so they are not stored in the body as fat.

"Grew by our feeding to so great a bulk" [101]

There are a few people who, in order to diminish body fat, choose to plunge into physical activity and use exercise as the exclusive method of reducing fat. Using exercise alone or using diet alone to try to reduce body fat is usually ineffective, difficult and may well be a waste of time. These misconceptions are commonly practiced and widely held. A reasonable and sound weight loss goal should be to lose approximately one pound of body fat per week.

97	King Lear, Act III, Sc. II
98	Romeo and Juliet, Act V, Sc. I
99	King John, Act V, Sc. VII
100	The Taming of the Shrew, Act II, Sc. I
101	King Henry IV, part I, Act V, Sc. I

"So, so; now sit: and look you eat no more" [102]

Before considering a weight loss program we must understand how the body uses the energy that is derived from the foods we eat each day. About seventy-five percent of the food energy that we eat, digest and have available in the body will be utilized preserving life and maintaining body functions such as respiration, circulation, building and repairing body cells, and maintaining body temperature. **"If I dare eat, or drink, or breathe, or live ... "** [103] In fact, as much as ten percent of the energy a person expends each day is spent by the body simply digesting and processing the food that was eaten.

"Time hath not yet so dried this blood of mine, Nor age so eat up" [104]

As we grow older, the amount of energy expended on life processes diminishes slightly, about a two percent decline each decade. This slowing of energy consumption is certainly a contributing factor to our ever-increasing body fat as we get older.

"To gorge his appetite" [105]

We live at a time and under circumstances in which eating is easy and therefore energy is plentiful. This presents us with the lifelong problem of avoiding excess and unnecessary energy consumption and eliminating needless energy that we munch our way through.

"I will desire you to live in the mean time, and eat your victuals: come, there is sauce for it." [106]

The vague and poorly understood, yet correct solution is exercise and activity. However, the problem is that even the most physically active lifestyle will use and eliminate only about twenty percent of the energy that we burn each day.

"Then feed, and be fat" [107]

What we must understand is that in order to eliminate body weight, say one pound of body fat, we need to expend three thousand five hundred calories. This being the amount of energy stored in a pound of body fat. This stored energy, fat, is not readily usable, or easily accessed. In order to accomplish this goal by simply eating less we would, at a minimum, have to reduce our daily food intake by at least five hundred calories every day—five hundred fewer calories everyday for seven days, therefore thirty-five hundred calories less per week. Five hundred fewer calories everyday, every week, every month not only would deprive us of needed energy but many essential nutrients as well. An additional

---

102   Titus Andronicus, Act III, Sc. II
103   King Richard II, Act IV, Sc. I
104   Much Ado About Nothing, Act IV, Sc. I
105   King Lear, Act I, Sc. I
106   King Henry V, Act V, Sc. I
107   King Henry Iv, part I, Act II, Sc. IV

problem arises when we consider that just eating less really does not demand the body to use stored energy, in fact quite the opposite is true. When one drastically reduces the amount of food (calories) consumed for weight loss reasons, the body does not realize that we are trying to intentionally lose weight. In fact, as a result of evolutionary survival mechanisms, the body responds to decreased food intake by attempting to conserve and preserve stored body fat by slowing down metabolic processes, and by minimizing all the body's energy expenditures. The body interprets our reduced food intake as a *famine* and attempts to survive and maintain life by protecting and preserving stored body energy, FAT. The "preserved" energy from FAT would be available for life processes in the days, weeks, and possibly even months of famine to come.

"tender preservation of our person" [108]

By contrast, weight loss efforts that involve exercise almost exclusively with no adjustment in eating are equally unsound. If we try to exercise vigorously for thirty minutes or more, we would have great difficulty in consuming or diminishing five hundred calories of stored energy. Exercise that is truly vigorous consumes, at the most, perhaps fifteen calories per minute and cannot be sustained for much more than just a few minutes, several at the most. If we try to moderate the intensity of the exercise so that we can continue for a longer period of time in order to meet our goal of losing one pound of body fat, we would have to swim approximately eight and a half miles or run the equivalent of about thirty-five miles every day.

"time and the hour runs through the roughest day"[109]

From these exercise extremes it should become obvious that choosing exercise only as the method of weight loss will result in only a few dozen, perhaps as many as a hundred extra calories being used. Truly vigorous exercise cannot be sustained or extended long enough on a regular basis to burn the hundreds of calories necessary to diminish body fat at a rate of a pound a week.

"A solemn combination shall be made"[110]

A combination of moderately intense, long duration physical activity and a reduced caloric, balanced diet, are essential for anyone who desires and seeks **"life, with grace, health, and beauty"**[111] as well as an improved body composition. The duration and intensity of the physical activity determines whether the body will use fat or carbohydrates as fuel during the activity. Moderately intense activity that is continuous for twenty minutes or more is the type of activity that will lead to stored body fat being reduced in the body as it is burned by the muscles.

---

108   King Henry V, Act II, Sc. II
109   Macbeth, Act I, Sc. III
110   Twelfth Night, Act V, Sc. I
111   King Lear, Act I, Sc. I

"How poor are they that have not patience!"[112]

A diet that severely restricts or denies a wide variety of foods or extremely low-calorie diets are usually ineffective and sometimes life threatening. It is essential that we take a long-range view of our weight loss goals. If we are going to be successful, it is obvious that we must combine appropriate exercise and a decreased caloric intake. Daily regular exercise at a reasonably intense level should expend about three hundred calories a day and is a reasonable goal. At the same time eating less, about two hundred fewer calories, would contribute to the reduction of about one pound of stored body fat each week. The key concept here is a moderate approach, one that reduces energy intake slightly, and increases energy expenditures slightly. Through this approach, the reduction, of approximately one pound of body fat per week is a reasonable, attainable goal. For most of us obsessed with and desiring rapid weight loss, these recommendations usually seem too slow.

"Till then, in patience our proceeding be."[113]

However, it has been shown that these procedures allow the body to lose weight gradually and systematically; preserve nutritional health; contribute to lean body maintenance and the weight is more likely to stay off. It allows you to modify your diet and activity levels in sensible increments and thus the prospect for quality living and sensible eating habits becomes more likely.

Diet plans that do not include physical activity are unsound. It is well understood that the excess body fat so common in modern society today, is as much the result of our inactive lifestyles, as it is our overeating. Attempting to **"make less thy body"**[114] and **"hence, ... more thy grace"**[115] by losing weight while living a sedentary life means living hungry, like a **"mountain of mad flesh."**[116] Achieving and maintaining a desirable and healthy amount of body fat is much more likely to be achieved if we combine healthy, slightly reduced eating with regular brisk long duration physical activity.

---

112   Othello, Act II, Sc. III
113   Hamlet, Act V, Sc. I
114   Henry IV, part II, Act V, Sc. V
115   Henry IV, part II, Act V, Sc. V
116   The Comedy of Errors, Act IV, Sc. IV

The Effect of This Good Lesson

Chapter VI

SHAKESPEAREAN FITNESS ADVICE

"I shall the effect of this good lesson keep" [1]

Physical fitness is replete with all manner of myth and misinformation. Despite all the well known benefits of regular physical activity, most people in today's **"very soft society"**[2] remain far too sedentary for their own good and their own health. Reasons and excuses for avoiding activity and exertion abound. In addition to widespread misinformation, weariness, boredom, and a lack of time are all common excuses which people use to justify their avoidance of physical activity and exercise. By contrast, we rarely feel the need to justify and have no difficulty finding the time to spend watching television or shopping. The basic fact is that there is no magic!

"The adage must be verified."[3]

The principles and practices that contribute to physical fitness have been known for many years. These truths include the same common sense activities and advice that has been around for decades. The difficulty is not in knowing them but rather incorporating them into our daily lives.

GENERAL FITNESS PRECEPTS

"Our bodies are our gardens, to the which our wills are gardeners"[4]

Achieving physical fitness requires a commitment of mind and body. Excuses are common and easy, and in modern society often get in the way of our pursuit of physical fitness. **"I know that. . . .it is fit I should commit."**[5] Fitness can be achieved but the obligation and the responsibility is ours. To achieve physical fitness we must make a lifestyle commitment to ourselves.

---

1 Hamlet, Act I, Sc. III
2 Hamlet, Act V, Sc. II
3 King Henry VI, part III, Act I, Sc. IV
4 Othello, Act I, Sc. III
5 Cymbeline, Act II, Sc. I

"let your own discretion be your tutor: suit the action to the word, the word to the action"[6]

It can be done! Take control and be prepared for one of the most healthful, beneficial experiences of life.

"No news but health from their physicians"[7]

𝕮onsult a physician before beginning an exercise program. Exercise deserves serious preparation and planning. This is especially true as **"haggish age steal[s] on."** [8] A physician can determine exercise suitability, general health and determine the safest and most effective exercise activities. Additionally, a physician can ascertain and advise of activities that may be undesirable or harmful.

"patience to you, and be well contented"[9]

We should proceed to our fitness goals patiently. We should progress slowly, and realistically. Going slower often results in getting there sooner. We must understand that physical improvements, diet and weight loss will occasionally plateau. These pauses or delays are temporary. We should not lose focus or commitment. **"Ambition should be made of sterner stuff."**[10] When these delays occur, we should simply maintain our dietary focus and active lifestyle and improvement will eventually resume. As we continue to pursue physical fitness, every few weeks we should intensify our efforts by increasing the frequency, duration, or intensity of activity. Progress will go on if we continue to challenge ourselves.

"aspiration lifts him from the earth"[11]

𝕿he quest for improved fitness, or for its maintenance, should begin gradually. **"Though this be all, do not so quickly go."** [12] We must not attempt to do too much too soon. We should set reasonable and attainable fitness goals. Reasonable short-term and long-term goals are essential if we are going to be successful in our pursuit of fitness. It is the key to success. Achievement of reasonable short-term goals will make it more likely that we may achieve long-term goals. **"Successively from age to age ... built it."** [13] As <u>physical fitness </u>improves, gradually push back existing physiological barriers and move

6	Hamlet, Act, III, Sc. II
7	Sonnet CXL
8	All's Well that Ends Well, Act I, Sc. II
9	King Henry VIII, Act V, Sc. I
10	Julius Caesar, Act III, Sc. II
11	Troilus and Cressida, Act IV, Sc. V
12	King Richard II, Act I, Sc. II
13	King Richard III, Act III, Sc. I

fitness goals to newer and higher levels. Let success be the motivator that leads to even higher achievement.

"I am constant to my purpose."[14]

With virtually all of the components of physical fitness, the healthiest, most effective, and best way to proceed is gradually.

"Not yet enjoy'd: so tedious is this day" [15]

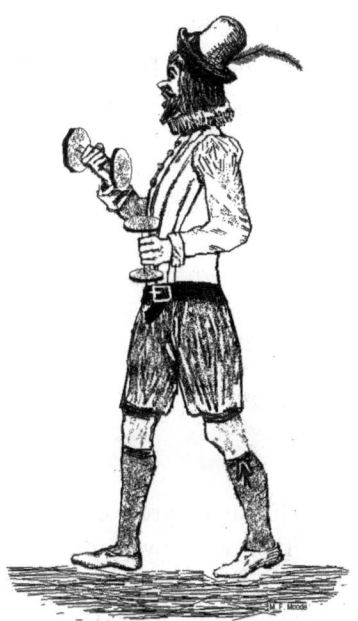

Move beyond the simple, somewhat shallow goals of just losing weight or increasing muscle strength and strive for *physical fitness*. Enjoy the physical activity **"so pleasure and action make the hours seem short."** [16] Focus on the present, and enjoy it! This ultimately will bring us more joy and lead to greater fitness achievements. We must stay committed to our long-term fitness goals but not let them become the source of agony or disappointment. Focusing on what we want to be or look like at some distant point in the future, when our exercise and dieting programs are over, may tend to discourage us and interfere with the progress we are currently making. The benefits of a sound fitness program are not spectacular or instantaneous and concentrating on our expectations of the future may make us lose sight of the present, and progress and benefits that have been achieved.

"Observe degree, priority and place" [17]

We should prioritize our fitness efforts in order to successfully meet the demands of life, work, family, and health. We rarely lack time. We do however waste it. We should try to make our exercise activities a high priority but not necessarily the most important aspect of life.

---

14   Hamlet, Act V, Sc. II
15   Romeo and Juliet, Act III, Sc. II
16   Othello, Act II, Sc. III
17   Troilus and Cressida, Act I, Sc. III

Physical Activity Admonitions
"With good advice and little medicine" [18]

"And ceremoniously let us prepare"[19]

Always prepare for exercise and fitness activities by undergoing a warm-up. Soft tissue injury is a possibility even if our form of activity is walking. The best way to avoid injury is to spend approximately five minutes moving at a steady, comfortable pace until our muscles are warm and we are just beginning to sweat. **"Now are we well prepared to know the pleasure"**[20] of exercise and physical activity. Following exercise, cool-down by reducing your activity effort gradually. Perform stretches and drink water. Because our muscles are warm from activity, this is an excellent time to stretch. These two procedures combined, warm-up and cool down, help to prevent injuries, facilitate recovery and are almost as important as exercising. When exercising, we should always allow enough time so we are not rushed and are able to include the warm-up and cool-down procedure.

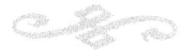

"Is he so young a man and so old a lifter?" [21]

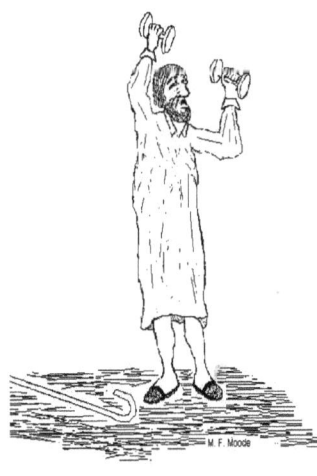

It is a common misconception that as we grow older our muscles shrink and turn to fat. This not only is untrue it is virtually impossible. One type of tissue cannot turn into another! Additionally, the passage of time, aging, does not necessarily cause muscle atrophy or fat gains. We know that regular physical activity along with a nutritious diet can maintain muscle function as well as muscle mass. A sensible active lifestyle will prevent undesirable body composition changes and maintain normal healthy muscle. Finally, even **"when service should in my old limbs lie lame"** [22] it is possible for a person, through exercise, aerobic activity, muscle work and a sound diet, to renew strength, increase mobility, reinforce bones and maintain flexibility.

---

18   King Henry IV, part II, Act III, Sc. I
19   The Merchant of Venice, Act V, Sc. I
20   King Henry V, Act I, Sc. II
21   Troilus and Cressida Act I, Sc. II
22   As You Like It, Act II, Sc. III

"No profit grows where is no pleasure ta'en
In brief, sir, study what you most affect"[23]

Choosing and performing activities we enjoy is an important first step toward reaching our fitness goals. Those we select should be pleasurable, easy to engage in, and fit comfortably into our lives.

"so long as nature Will bear up with this exercise,
so long I daily vow to use it."[24]

Whether it is aerobic classes, jogging, walking, or riding a bike we should choose activities we look forward to doing and can regularly and often pursue.

"By taking nor by giving of excess"[25]

To reduce body fat we should reduce our caloric intake a little and moderately increase our caloric expenditures. That is, we should eat a little less and try to be a bit more physically active. It is not necessary to engage in physical activity and exercise constantly and at all times to reduce body fat. In order to expend more calories, live a physically active lifestyle and engage in enjoyable activities whenever we can. Walking, biking or swimming for thirty minutes or more at least five times a week would be an appropriate and positive way to begin a physical fitness activity program. This procedure may seem overly simple and painfully slow at first, but the fat will diminish with time and the body will adapt and improve.

"And you shall see 'tis purchased by the weight"[26]

Weightlifting exercises are best suited for the improvement of muscle strength, endurance, or both. Muscles, when they are regularly used, increase the body's metabolic rate, which may indirectly help diminish body fat. Increased metabolism enhances the number of calories we expend at rest and while active. Weightlifting will condition our body cells to become more effective energy consumers and body fat reducers. This higher rate of energy consumption occurs continuously, all day, all night, at rest and at work.

---

23   The Taming of the Shrew, Act I, Sc. I
24   The Winter's Tale, Act III, Sc. II
25   The Merchant of Venice Act I, Sc. III
26   The Merchant of Venice, Act III, Sc. II

"Thereby to see the minutes how they run"[27]

The way to reduce body fat is to expend more energy than we consume. Activities as simple as walking, biking or swimming will suffice. More important than the activity is the duration and frequency that we spend engaged in the activity. Thirty minutes or more, five times a week is a sound initial approach to weight loss through exercise. Weight loss under all circumstances is a slow process but once the process begins it can continue as long as the lifestyle is maintained.

"they have conjoin'd all three"[28]

A sound exercise program should include aerobic activity, resistance training and sound nutrition. An understanding of these three aspects of fitness is essential for enhancing physical fitness and the functioning of the heart and lungs, as well as improved nutrient delivery to all body cells. Additionally, the most prevalent body component, muscle, is effectively worked and the nutritionally sound diet ensures health, function and maintenance.

"what hast thou then more than thou hadst before?"[29]

Fitness contributes to more than just quality of life, physical abilities, and general well being. Being physically fit can facilitate health. It strengthens the immune system, reduces the risk of cardiovascular diseases, skeletal and postural difficulties, certain cancers as well as diseases related to obesity and excess body fat. Additionally, fitness may enhance and improve our social attitudes, family interactions, and work commitments. Ultimately, a fitness lifestyle can reduce the effects of aging as well as the adverse effects of stress which characterize so much of modern life.

"Assemble presently the people hither"[30]

Exercising regularly with others or being part of a fitness group or a fitness class can help us maintain our motivation and reinforces our personal commitment. It is much easier to

27 King Henry VI, part III, Act II Sc. V
28 A Midsummer Night's Dream, Act III, Sc. II
29 Sonnet XL
30 Coriolanus, Act III, Sc. III

skip an exercise session when we are on our own. When we have an obligation to others we are more likely to follow through with our commitments. Having fitness friends may be just what we need.

"to be used according to your state" [31]

"**When fitness calls them on**" [32] exercise and physical activity should not be a competitive endeavor. Rather, fitness activities should be performed at our own pace and at an intensity level that is comfortable and reflects our personal state of physical condition. **"More than a little is by much too much."** [33] It is unsound and wrong to be competitive as a part of a fitness program.

"Thy pains not used must by thyself be paid" [34]

Physical activity and exercise should not be painful! The old cliché *"no gain without pain"* is not true. There is a significant difference between soreness and pain. Soreness is not unusual when we begin an exercise program, but the body adapts quickly and soreness should disappear promptly as we become more fit. Pain associated with physical activity is usually an indication that we are doing something wrong. If we are experiencing pain, our exercise is either too severe, too intense, or being performed incorrectly. If we are finding it difficult to complete our normal exercise routine on any given day, we should slow down or stop. We should never ignore exercise-related pain.

"filed with my abilities: mine own ends" [35]

Normative tables, charts, predictive graphs are all fine and interesting, however we should set our physical fitness goals based on ourselves, how we feel, and how fit we are. The challenge is to become as good as we are able to be. To strive to achieve or compete with goals and standards that are derived from huge populations that only exist in some statistical world is not a fair measurement of our fitness abilities. Our real and measured performances and abilities should be our motivation rather than statistical abstractions.

31	King Henry VI, part II, Act II Sc. IV
32	Troilus and Cressida Act I, Sc. III
33	King Henry IV, part I, Act III, Sc. I
34	Alls Well That Ends Well, Act II, Sc. I
35	King Henry VII, Act III, Sc. II

"And to thy worth will add right worthy gains" [36]

When we begin an exercise regimen, it is not unusual to experience slight weight gains. These weight gains may be the result of increasing muscle mass. Even while losing body fat, body weight may not change as quickly as we desire or expect. This because changes in body composition, whether increases in one component or decreases in another, do not occur at the same rate. Additionally, the body may be changing in ways we are not even expecting. We may be losing inches in body girth, increasing muscle tone, and increasing muscle size. The key is be patient and not to be overly preoccupied with conspicuous visible results. Ultimately, desirable body composition changes will occur.

"I am a simple woman, much too weak" [37]

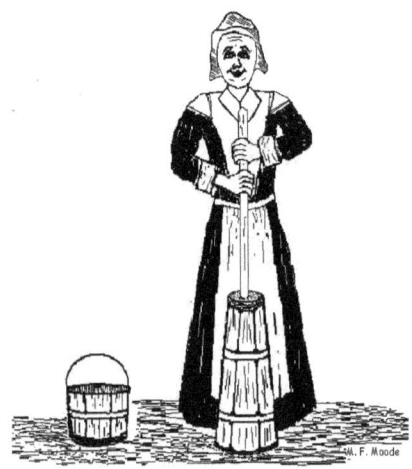

There exists a common misconception that women who exercise regularly with weights will develop masculine physiques as their muscles will, just like men's, continue to get bigger and bigger. The tendency to develop big muscles is gender related and it is virtually impossible for women to develop large muscles similar to a man's. Apart from the genetics, women lack the hormones necessary to develop massive muscular physiques, **"women, being the weaker vessels."** [38]

A women's shape may change and she may gain some weight by using weights in her physical fitness programs. Generally though, **"women are soft, mild ... and flexible"** [39] and weight lifting will be effective and beneficial for developing muscle tone and improving muscle strength and endurance, if not muscle size.

---

36   King Richard II, Act V, Sc. VI
37   King Henry VIII, Act II, Sc. IV
38   Romeo and Juliet, Act I Sc. I
39   King Henry VI, part III, Act I, Sc. IV

The Effect of This Good Lesson

"Whilst, like a willing patient, I will drink" [40]

When exercising, we must replenish body fluids before we feel thirsty. **"Water to quench it."** [41] By the time thirst has risen to the level of consciousness we are probably already dehydrated and performance will be adversely affected. One of the byproducts of the physical work is heat which is produced in the muscles. This heat causes body temperature to rise. Heat is transported by the blood from muscles to the skin where perspiration is formed and hopefully evaporates thus dissipating heat and maintaining a reasonable body temperature. As activity continues, unless water is constantly being replaced, it is possible to become dangerously dehydrated.

"Health and fair time of day; joy and good wishes" [42]

It is a common belief that morning exercise increases our energy level and gets our day started with vigor. Conversely, it is a common misconception that exercise at night may lead to restlessness and hinder sleep. The truth is that there is no best time to exercise and whatever time we are used to will probably be right for us. Usually the time we have to exercise is a matter of convenience. The most important thing is to include physical activity and exercise into our lives whenever it is convenient.

"As sure as his guts are made of puddings" [43]

Performing sit-ups, crunches, or any other exercises directed at the abdominal region probably will not reduce fat in that area, or guarantee a flat stomach or prominent abdominal musculature. While sit-ups and crunches can improve abdominal muscle endurance and occasionally strengthen abdominal muscles, these exercises do not burn the fat that is stored immediately under the skin of the abdomen. To burn fat and flatten our **"fair round belly,"** [44] we need to

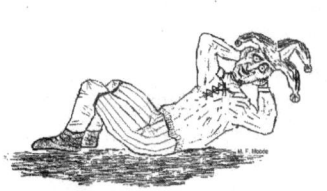

40	Sonnet CXI
41	Coriolanus Act V Sc. II
42	King Henry V, Act V, Sc. II
43	Merry Wives of Windsor, Act II, Sc. I
44	As You Like It, Act II, Sc. VII

consume the stored fat energy through long duration, moderately intense activity. Sit-ups, crunches, and other similar abdominal exercises are not capable of being performed for a long enough time nor are they sufficiently intense to reduce stored fat. Because muscles in a particular area are active, this does not mean that fat stored in that area is being reduced. Fat is utilized in the body in a general way, coming from all over, with the most recently stored fat being utilized first! If we engage in appropriately vigorous activity for a sufficient amount of time, fat from all over the body, including the abdomen, will be diminished.

Once we have eliminated the fat, our stomach muscles will be more visible. Many fitness experts believe that our preoccupation with abdominal musculature may hinder digestion and interfere with the diaphragm and breathing. That is, with regard to abdominal muscles, we should **"scant this excess"** [45] and have as our goal a toned but relaxed abdomen rather than taunt and prominent muscles. It is an interesting contradiction that washboard abs are often considered desirable and attractive; while this type of abdominal musculature may be undesirable and unhealthy. The development of abdominal muscles through **"the immoderate use** [of abdominal exercises] **turns to restraint"** [46] and may lead to misalignment of the spine and serious back pain.

"Swell'st thou, proud heart? i'll give thee scope to beat" [47]

If our exercise objective is to reduce body fat, then we should engage in exercise or perform fitness activities that are within our predetermined exercise heart rate range. It is possible, and not that uncommon, to work too hard at reducing fat—to engage in exercise so intense that the body consumes energy in the muscles, energy in the blood and not energy stored as body fat.

"Why tell you me of moderation?" [48]

When performing moderately intense aerobic activity the body has the need and the time to convert and consume the stored energy of the body—fat. When we exercise excessively hard, beyond the predetermined exercise heart rate, the body cannot get the oxygen necessary to effectively burn stored body fat. Aerobic activity, performed within the predetermined exercise heart rate, means our muscles are working in an oxygen-rich environment which is conducive to using and diminishing stored body fat. After approximately twenty minutes of aerobic activity the body achieves a steady state (homeostasis) at which point energy demands and energy production are about equal. Physical activity performed at a moderately high level of homeostasis may continue for a very long time. When this happens, the body will probably utilize fat as its source of energy.

---

45   The Merchant of Venice, Act III, Sc. II
46   Measure Fore Measure, Act I, Sc. II
47   King Richard II, Act III, Sc. III
48   Troilus and Cressida, Act IV, Sc. IV

The Effect of This Good Lesson

"How light and portable my pain seems now" 49

𝕵oint pain which results from some forms of arthritis can be diminished by keeping joints movable and active. An excellent physical activity for maintaining or improving bone and joint health is swimming. This because water supports body weight, massages limbs and is not an impact type of activity. Thus exercising in water can be a factor in skeletal improvement, joint health, and enhanced flexibility without causing pain or putting undo stress on arthritic joints.

"… . health and living now begins to mend" 50

𝕿o improve or maintain physical fitness we simply need to get started, and as the commercial advises *just do it*. The desire to improve is most likely to succeed when it is internally motivated. **"… . then begins a journey in my head."** 51 If, however, we tell ourselves we need somebody's assistance or something external, or outside of our own self-determination to get us into an exercise mode, we will probably fail or put off beginning or continuing an exercise program. Having a partner or friends to exercise with makes the experience more enjoyable and one is more likely to continue and succeed. However, there are those who believe that a professional trainer to lead, motivate and guide the conditioning experience is a necessity. This belief is false, and many professional fitness trainers are little more than exercise, lap, or repetition counters, that make their living on individuals who believe they need outside motivation.

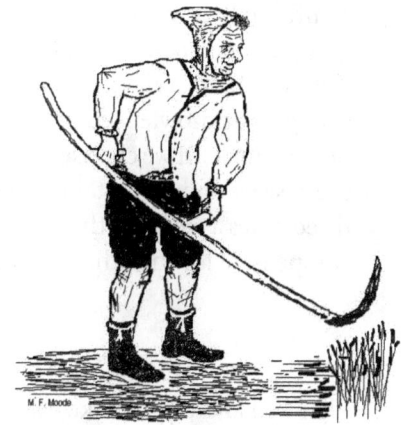

"A little riper and more lusty" 52

𝕴f we take responsibility for our physical activity and practice sound nutrition, we can redefine the modern concept of aging. A person is never too old to begin a physical fitness

---

49	King Lear, Act III, Sc. VI
50	Timon of Athens, Act V, Sc. I
51	Sonnet XXVII
52	As You Like It, Act III, Sc. V

program or benefit from physical activity. We do however, **"in the idle pleasures of these days"** [53] frequently ignore and neglect the benefits and advantages of physical activity **"and as with age ... [the] body uglier grow[s]."** [54] The value of fitness includes a longer life, improved health, positive attitude and a brighter more positive disposition. Fitness types of exercise means moving the body in ways that increases oxygen demands, blood flow, and muscle activity for reasonably long periods of time.

"in what motion age will give me leave" [55]

"He that shall live this day, and see old age" [56] if able to walk should be able to exercise. If walking is difficult or limited we can begin an exercise program by moving or lifting our legs. Many people who believe they are too old to exercise have never engaged in physical activity and probably do not understand the concept, procedures, or benefits.

"You are too blunt: go to it orderly." [57]

Performing exercises or working-out on an *irregular* basis, whether slowly and comfortably or vigorously is not sound, does not contribute effectively to fitness, and may well put a person at risk of injury. A regular and orderly approach to exercise is essential if it is to be of value. An exercise routine of three thirty-minute work-outs per week is generally acknowledged to be the absolute minimum activity that will contribute to fitness maintenance. If we choose, or are forced to pursue fitness through this minimal approach to exercise we should certainly supplement it by living a physically active lifestyle. Exercising three times a week for thirty minutes,—an hour and a half of exercise, does not and will not compensate for the other one hundred sixty six and a half hours which are left in a week.

".... make it orderly and well,
According to the fashion and the time." [58]

Plan well and try to make exercise as convenient as possible. The body does not care where the activity demand comes from—it will respond. The activity demands may be from weights, gymnasium equipment, exercise equipment, physical work or any manner of work-out devices.

---

53 King Richard III, Act I, Sc. I
54 The Tempest, Act IV, Sc. I
55 All's Well that Ends Well, Act II, Sc. III
56 King Henry V, Act IV, Sc. III
57 The Taming of the Shrew, Act II, Sc. I
58 The Taming of the Shrew, Act IV, Sc. III

Nutrition, Diet, and Body Composition

"For food and diet, to some enterprise That hath a stomach in't" [59]

It is very likely that a day will come when we recognize that we have lost our youthful physiques and gained unwanted weight. The common reaction is to begin a diet. This response, is an attempt to diminish stored body fat all over the body by reducing the nutrients we put in our mouths! This is not only unsound it is illogical and often ineffective. The one action does not necessarily or permanently lead to the desired result. The concept of "*diet*" is very common in modern society and unfortunately is very narrow, misguided and sets us up for disappointment and failure. To reduce body fat and lose weight it would be far better to consider fat reduction and weight-loss as a lifestyle approach which includes nutritious eating as well as an appropriate purposeful physically active lifestyle. To conclude, we must be clear about our weight loss goals. It is far more appropriate and sound to strive toward being physically fit and energetic than it is to pursue simply **"a lean and hungry look."** [60]

"Your greatest want is, you want much of meat." [61]

There is a belief that the greater the exercise, the more protein there should be in the diet. This simply is not true! It is not necessary or desirable to increase the amount of protein in our daily diet when we engage in regular exercise.

"What, are there but three?" [62]

Of the three energy nutrients, protein, carbohydrate and fat, protein is the least desirable and least efficient energy source. Carbohydrates are the best source of muscle energy. Fats are a good source of energy but an extremely complicated source of energy for the body to access and utilize. Protein is necessary for building body tissue, maintenance of cell and physiological system integrity, as well as general body repairs.

59	Hamlet, Act I, Sc. I
60	Julius Caesar, Act I, Sc. II
61	Timon of Athens, Act IV, Sc. III
62	Love's Labour's Lost, Act V, Sc. II

Arise Forth from the Couch: A Shakespearean Guide to Physical Fitness

"Sir, sooth to say, you did not dine at home" [63]

Today it is common to dine out almost as often as we prepare our own meals. We should try whenever possible to avoid fast food restaurants. Dining out should not be an excuse or the cause of eating unhealthy, excessively, or poorly. Take the time and make the effort to eat nutritionally balanced and healthy meals. A simple guide to healthy eating would be to avoid anything served in a box, a bag, or wrapped in paper. Additionally, anything that is served to you through a car window is probably nutritionally a **"loathed choice".** [64] One other simple eating guideline might be to never eat anything that would probably not have been present on a restaurant menu one hundred years ago. **"To hear good counsel: o, what learning is."** [65] Fast foods are characteristically too high in fat, salt, sugar and calories. They are, however, convenient, cheap, and are pleasing to the taste. These types of foods are simply **"inventions to delight the taste"** [66] and serve few, if any, nutritional needs. Fast food eaten regularly undermines health, **"the outward composition of. . . . [the] body"** [67] and detracts from our general well-being. The body's nutritional demands should not be fulfilled primarily through fast food dining. Try to spend whatever time and effort is necessary to have nutritious foods, prepared and served as simply as possible and in wholesome appropriate quantities.

"Be bounteous at our meal." [68]

A sound nutritious diet is essential for health and wellness and must not be neglected when attempting to change body composition and lose weight. To **"forbear, and eat no more,"** [69] skip meals, or load meals in favor of one or more food types or at the expense of various nutritional groups or food kinds is unsound and unhealthy. We must understand there is no magic! We should not believe in or take diet potions or exotic combinations of foods, or nutritional additives, and diet supplements. Avoid fad diets or impractical eating plans. The best approach to eating is **"to breakfast with what appetite you have."** [70] After breakfast, and a morning of sensible physical activity **"then to dinner."** [71] Finally, as the day wanes **"to that nourishment which is called supper"** [72] but with the

---

63	The Comedy of Errors, Act IV, Sc. IV
64	Titus Andronicus, Act, IV Sc. II
65	Romeo and Juliet, Act III, Sc. III
66	Pericles, Prince of Tyre Act I, Sc. IV
67	King Henry VI, part I, Act II, Sc. III
68	Antony and Cleopatra, Act IV, Sc. II
69	As You Like It, Act II, Sc. VII
70	King Henry VIII Act III, Sc. II
71	The Taming of the Shrew, Act II, Sc. I.
72	Love's Labour's Lost, Act I, Sc. I

knowledge that during and **"between our after-supper and bed-time"**[73] desserts, sweets or as in Elizabethan times **"anchovies and sack after supper"** [74] should be avoided.

"the heavens have shaped my body so" [75]

We all inherit genetic tendencies which predetermine the range within which our body's size, shape, and type will develop. Unfortunately many of us in our **"present time's so sick"** [76] live our lives on the negative and undesirable side of our genetic potential. Though we may be getting taller from generation to generation, we also are wearing far more fat than we should under our skin, around our waists, on our thighs, hips, abdomen, and *butts*. Understanding and appreciating our genetic inheritance can contribute to the likelihood that we may achieve our maximum potential rather than fall short or possibly even pursue unattainable goals. It is our modern sedentary lifestyle's that contributes most to our present-day tendency to become progressively fatter from generation to generation. Though genetic inheritance plays an important role, it does not determine what we have for dinner or how often we exercise.

"A man who for this three months hath not. . . .taken sustenance" [77]

Food deprivation, starvation, and crash dieting are unsound, and dangerous ways to diet and do not work. **"And give them life whom hunger starved half dead."** [78] When we live our lives with severely restricted diets, our metabolism slows down, making it less likely that we will lose weight. Sudden or severe food restriction triggers the body's survival mechanisms. The body goes into "survival mode," trying to preserve energy in order to maintain life as long as possible.

"Now can I break my fast, dine, sup and sleep" [79]

Rapid weight loss is often a sign that the diet being used is unhealthy. Additionally, using diet drugs, herbs, and the latest weight loss potions is dangerous. Making slow, gradual changes in the amount of stored body fat gives the body time to adjust to the new physical changes that normally occur with sound healthy weight reduction procedures.

73	A Midsummer Night's Dream, Act V, Sc. I
74	King Henry IV, part I, Act II, Sc. IV
75	King Henry VI, part III, Act V, Sc. VI
76	King John, Act V, Sc. I
77	Pericles, Prince of Tyre, Act V, Sc. I
78	Pericles, Prince of Tyre, Act I, Sc. IV
79	The Two Gentlemen of Verona, Act II, Sc. IV

"With lesser weight but not with lesser woe" [80]

Using a scale to gauge weight loss progress is not a sound or accurate means of evaluating progress. A scale cannot distinguish between fat and lean body mass. It is, in fact, possible to lose fat and gain weight. Similarly, it is possible to lose weight and not lose fat. This could occur because of an increase in muscle mass if regular systematic exercise is a major part of our weight loss program.

"look how well my garments sit upon me" [81]

Weight loss may be reasonably monitored by the way our clothes fit. We should keep and try on some of our out-grown old clothes to see how they fit. Weight loss progress may be immediately appreciated if our old clothes are loose, conversely weight gains may be noticed if these clothes are becoming even smaller.

"Shall I be tempted to infringe my vow" [82]

Eating appropriately nutritious reasonably reduced calorie meals in order to decrease excess body fat takes a long-term commitment. Therefore, " **... fix most firm thy resolution**" [83] and pursue weight loss goals slowly. At the same time, we must be aware that depriving ourselves of the foods we enjoy may lead to frustration and undermine our progress. It is acceptable to allow ourselves to enjoy from time to time the pleasure of foods we particularly like. This can and should be done freely and without a guilty conscience. This is especially true if physical activity is a regular part of our weight loss diet program. It is always possible to compensate for these indulgences by working out a little longer or by making small changes to our subsequent eating to balance energy intake.

"the taste confounds the appetite" [84]

We should give careful consideration to what we eat, how it is prepared, and how it is served. Eating should not be motivated simply by pleasing tastes. **"Cloy the hungry**

80	The Comedy of Errors Act I Sc. I	
81	The Tempest Act II, Sc. I	
82	Coriolanus, Act V, Sc. III	
83	Othello, Act V, Sc.I	
84	Romeo and Juliet Act II, Sc. VI	

edge of appetite." [85] Focus on the need to eat healthy, wholesome, well prepared meals. Foods prepared by broiling, boiling, baking, braising or barbeque grilling are good choices that can contribute to a nutritious diet.

"feed on nourishing dishes." [86]

Further we must pay attention to the body's signs of hunger and fullness. It usually takes some time for the body to realize that it is satisfied, allow about twenty minutes after eating before considering second helpings. The body's nutritional and energy needs should determine our food intake, not cravings, pleasing tastes, emotions or moods.

"I'll make you feed on berries and on roots" [87]

𝕴ruits and vegetables are healthy and well known to be nutritionally rich sources of carbohydrates, vitamins, minerals, fiber, anti-oxidants, as well as good sources of energy.

"And I think the word sallet[88] was born to do me good. . . ." [89]

Additionally, it is common knowledge that good nutrition and healthy eating should include plenty of fruits and vegetables. A simple application of this nutritional knowledge is to eat many servings of different colored fruits and vegetables every day. A problem does exist however, when, either because of personal preference or for the purpose of losing weight, we eat excessive amounts of fruits and vegetables at the expense of other food groups. **"Sir, I will eat no meat."** [90] Too many fruits and vegetables in the diet, especially if other nutrients are restricted are unhealthy and may put a person into a nutritional deficiency. This deficiency occurs, because fruits are water dense and rich in fiber while most vegetables are relatively low in calories. This combination allows the water to flush many nutrients out of the body and contributes to poor nutrition.

"We cannot live on grass, on berries, water, As beasts and birds and fishes. " [91]

Weight loss which results from this emphasis on fruits and vegetables is unsound and weight lost probably will not be permanent. Like any caloric restrictive diet, the fruit and vegetable approach may lead to reductions of lean body mass and considerable amounts of water loss. It is easier however, to get all of the nutrients the body needs for good health,

---

85	King Richard II, Act I, Sc. III
86	Othello, Act III, Sc. III
87	Titus Andronicus, Act IV, Sc. II
88	Salad
89	Henry VI, Act II, Sc. IV
90	Antony and Cleopatra, Act V, Sc. II
91	Timon of Athens, Act IV, Sc. III

optimal function, cell growth, muscle maintenance, and energy when meals contain a desirable blend of proteins, complex carbohydrates, and fats.

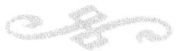

". . . . minister'st a potion unto me" [92]

Today, unscrupulous companies sell pills, potions, weight loss creams and numerous other products that claim to reduce body fat. Weight loss without physical activity is an extremely attractive concept in our sedentary society. Despite the outrageous claims made by manufacturers, there is little or no evidence to suggest that these creams are effective in promoting fat loss. **"With no rash potion"** [93] or miracle topical lotion will either fat be reduced or body composition improved. There are no short cuts. **"If it appear not plain and prove untrue,"** [94] we should not fall for it! There are no new, miracle fat reduction discoveries! Unprincipled entrepreneurs are making millions of dollars at the expense of those seeking weight loss magic. The way body fat should be reduced is by reducing energy consumption (eat less) and increase energy output (use muscles). Diet and weight loss claims that suggest results will be miraculous are certainly exaggerated, and definitely untrue. Additionally, none of the newly developed pharmaceuticals have any significant impact on reducing obesity. Some, such as Phen-Fen have resulted in death. Others have resulted in dependence and addiction or at the least intestinal discomfort. Drug companies and manufacturers of *nutritional supplements* are researching how they can generate massive profits by creating something that appears to aid weight loss. Whether it does or not is not particularly important.

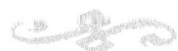

"To keep with you at meals, comfort your bed" [95]

It is a common misconception that eating immediately prior to going to bed at night will lead to a greater fat gain than if the same meal were consumed during the day. There is virtually no factual basis for this belief. Although eating late at night or snacking might be an unsound dietary habit, this practice does not result in a greater weight gain than if the same meal had been eaten at some other time during the day. The person who grows fatter is the person **"whose house, whose bed, whose meal[s], and exercise"** [96] are imbalanced, purposeless and flawed. Remember, it is our total daily caloric intake and energy expenditures that will determine if we gain fat, not the time of day that we eat.

---

92   Pericles, Prince of Tyre, Act I Sc. II
93   The Winter's Tale, Act I, Sc. II
94   All's Well That Ends Well, Act V, Sc. III
95   Julius Caesar, Act II Sc. I
96   Coriolanus, Act IV, Sc. IV

THE EFFECT OF THIS GOOD LESSON

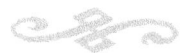

Epilogue

**"an epilogue or discourse, to make plain
Some obscure precedence that hath tofore been sain."** [97]

We should set our life goals beyond the basics. **"There are more things in heaven and earth"** [98] than just being physically fit and eating nutritionally well. These are just two aspects of human existence. Pursuing consciously and continually the highest level of well being should be our ultimate goal. It is not unusual to set our goals too low, inappropriately high and almost always too narrowly.

**"What a piece of work is man! How noble in reason!
How infinite in faculties! In form and moving, how
express and admirable! In action, how like an angel!
In apprehension, how like a god! The beauty of the world! The paragon of animals!"** [99]

The truly healthy, fit, and well individual should understand and practice good health, possess reasonable levels of physical fitness, pursue meaningful intellectual endeavors, work a satisfying and significant job, live a comfortable environmentally sound existence, recognize the spiritual aspects of humanity, and function in socially desirable and appropriate ways.

**"Proceed, proceed: we will begin these rites,
As we do trust they'll end, in true delights."** [100]

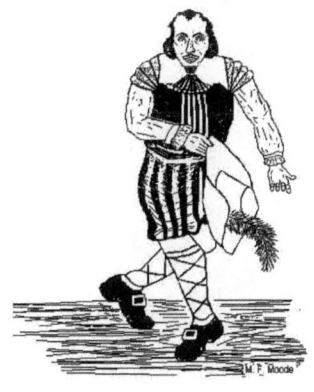

97	Love's Labour's Lost, Act III, Sc. I
98	Hamlet, Act I, Sc. V
99	Hamlet, Act II, Sc. II
100	As You Like It, Act V, Sc. IV

Selected Bibliography

The following are the principle books utilized in the preparation of this text.

Altoff, S. A., Svoboda, M., & Girdano, D. A. (3rd Edition) *Choices in Health and Fitness for Life.* Scottsdale, AZ, Gorsuch Scarisbrick, Publishers, 1996.

Asimov, Isaac. *Asimov's Guide to Shakespeare.* New York, NY, Avenel Books, 1978.

Biagioli, B.D., *Advanced Concepts of Personal Training.* South Miami, FL, NCSF Corporation. 2007.

Bloom, Harold. *Shakespeare The Invention of the Human.* New York, NY, Riverhead Books, 1998.

Boyce, Charles. *Shakespeare A To Z.* New York, NY, A Laurel Trade Paperback, 1990.

Bryson, Bill. *Shakespeare The World as Stage.* New York, NY Harper Collins Publishers, 2007.

Crystal, David and Crystal, Ben. *Shakespeare's Words A Glossary and Language Companion* Penguin, London, 2002.

Epstein, Norrie. *The Friendly Shakespeare.* New York, NY, Viking, 1993.

Edlin G., Golanty, E., & Brown K. M. (6th Edition). *Health and Wellness.* Sudsbury, MA, Jones and Bartlett Publishers, 1999.

Pinciss, G. M. and Lockyer, R. (eds.) *Shakespeare's World Background Readings in the English Renaissance.* New York, NY The Continuum Publishing Company, 1990

Prentice, W.E. (4th Edition). *Get Fit Stay Fit.* New York, NY, McGraw-Hill, 2001.

Staunton, Howard. (ed.) *The Complete Illustrated Shakespeare.* New York, NY, Gallery Books, 1989.

www.ingramcontent.com/pod-product-compliance
Lightning Source LLC
Chambersburg PA
CBHW080212040426
42333CB00043B/2554